Improving Support for America's Hidden Heroes

A RESEARCH BLUEPRINT

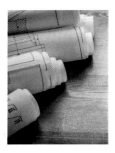

Terri Tanielian
Kathryn E. Bouskill
Rajeev Ramchand
Esther M. Friedman
Thomas E. Trail
Angela Clague

Sponsored by the Elizabeth Dole Foundation

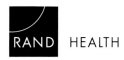

RAND HEALTH

For more information on this publication, visit www.rand.org/t/RR1873

Library of Congress Cataloging-in-Publication Data is available for this publication

ISBN: 978-0-8330-9767-5

Published by the RAND Corporation, Santa Monica, Calif.

© Copyright 2017 RAND Corporation

RAND® is a registered trademark.

Cover image: mihalec/GettyImages

Support RAND
Make a tax-deductible charitable contribution at
www.rand.org/giving/contribute

www.rand.org

Preface

In 2014, more than ten years after U.S. operations in Iraq and Afghanistan began and 2.7 million members of the armed forces were deployed, the RAND Corporation published *Hidden Heroes: Caring for Military Families*. The research, sponsored by the Elizabeth Dole Foundation, attracted significant attention to caregivers—typically, family members who provide significant aid to the country's wounded, ill, and injured service members by organizing and transporting them to their medical appointments; overseeing their finances; caring for their children; helping them relearn basic motor skills as necessary; and assisting them with their activities of daily living, such as eating, dressing, and bathing. *Hidden Heroes* documented the characteristics of the military and veteran caregiver population, offered insight on gaps in current programs, and provided recommendations to augment support for these caregivers. One such recommendation was to conduct additional research because the current literature on military and veteran caregivers is sparse. There have been several recent additions to the scholarly literature concerning caregivers' mental, physical, occupational, and financial hardships—that is, the burden that informal caregivers face; however, recognizing the adversity addresses only one aspect of the research needed to better support this population.

This study canvasses the research landscape on caregivers to identify strategic research needs for future investment. To achieve this objective, our RAND research team inventoried the currently available research on caregiving for disabled adults, children, and the elderly and gathered stakeholder input by conducting a survey and facilitating an online panel to allow a diverse set of stakeholders to voice their views on crucial topics for research. Based on a synthesis of this information, we devised a blueprint for future military and veteran caregiver research. The findings from this study will be of interest to researchers, stakeholders, and funders moving forward for future investment and collaboration in military and veteran caregiver research.

This report was sponsored by the Elizabeth Dole Foundation, and the research was conducted in RAND Health, a division of the RAND Corporation. A profile of RAND Health, abstracts of its publications, and ordering information can be found at www.rand.org/health.

Contents

Figures and Tables

Summary

In 2014, with funding support from the Elizabeth Dole Foundation, the RAND Corporation published *Hidden Heroes: America's Military Caregivers*, which shed light on the number and characteristics of, as well as the burden faced by, the estimated 5.5 million military and veteran caregivers who provide informal care and support to current and former U.S. service members (Ramchand, Tanielian, et al., 2014).[1] The study also offered recommendations for ensuring better support for these caregivers in the future. Among the recommendations was a call for additional research to improve understanding of how caregiver and care recipient needs evolve over time; how well specific programs for caregivers and care recipients are working; and how caregiving differentially affects specific subgroups, including children. The Elizabeth Dole Foundation asked RAND to develop a *research blueprint* to guide future investments that would improve the well-being of caregivers. The blueprint metaphor is useful for describing future caregiving research. Specifically,

- In the construction world, a *site plan* shows the footprint of the building on a lot, or how it fits onto a given space. In caregiving research, an analogous construct is *research that examines how caregiving and caregivers fit within the context of society at large.*
- A *floor plan* describes the relationships between rooms and spaces on one floor of the building. For caregiving research, an analogous construct is *research that examines the impacts of caregiving on caregivers, care recipients, and their families.*
- An *elevation* shows the building from the outside. In caregiving research, an analogous construct *is research that examines how external factors may influence caregiving.*

Assembling Expertise

We sought data from multiple sources and experts. Figure S.1 shows our overall approach.

---

[1] We use the term *military and veteran caregiver* to be inclusive of both those caring for a current member of the military (including active-duty, reserve, and National Guard members) and those caring for a former member of the military (commonly referred to as a veteran).

Figure S.1
Analytic Strategy

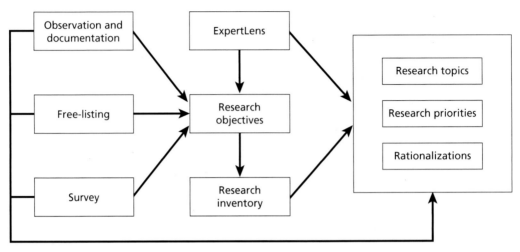

We took advantage of opportunities offered at the "Empowering Hidden Heroes: Pathways to InnoVAtion" summit, cosponsored by the Elizabeth Dole Foundation and the U.S. Department of Veterans Affairs, which took place in Washington, D.C., in September 2016. Attendees included the range of stakeholders whose input we sought: policy and program officials, government officials, researchers, clinicians, funders, advocates, care recipients, and caregivers. We attended multiple presentations and conducted a free-listing exercise that involved inviting attendees to generate research questions and priorities. In addition, we administered a survey to attendees to assess perceptions about specific priorities. Attendees included individuals and organizational representatives from the military and veteran caregiving stakeholder community specifically, as well as some representatives from the caregiving support community more broadly.

We integrated information from these sources to develop a list of caregiver-related research objectives. We then reviewed studies evaluating these objectives, looking at both military and veteran caregivers and informal caregivers more broadly. Finally, we used ExpertLens™—a RAND-developed, web-based tool that assesses stakeholder consensus—to elicit ratings of each research objective from panels of stakeholders that included representatives from the stakeholder groups listed above. We included three panels: one comprising military and veteran caregivers; one comprising caregiving researchers, government officials, and funders; and one comprising program leaders. The second and third groups included individuals from the military and veteran caregiver support community, as well as the caregiver support community more broadly.

Table S.1 lists the ten research objectives we developed, organized by major focus.

Table S.1
Research Objectives and Organization of the Blueprint

Blueprint Component	Focus	Research Objectives
Site plan	Caregivers as members of society	• Describe caregivers. • Quantify the societal cost savings attributed to caregiving.
Floor plan	Impacts of caregiving on caregivers, care recipients, and their families	• Document the effects of caregiving on caregiver outcomes. • Assess the consequences of caregiving on the children of caregivers. • Document the effects of caregiving on care recipient outcomes. • Assess how the needs of care recipients change over time. • Examine factors associated with caregiver and care recipient harm.
Elevation	External factors that influence caregiving	• Identify strategies for making effective programs available to more caregivers. • Evaluate the effectiveness of programs and policies for ensuring caregiver well-being. • Identify effective programs and policies to support caregivers' ability to provide care.

Describing Our Research Objectives

In this section, we describe each objective and summarize observations from our five data sources about the objective's importance, cultural acceptability, implementation cost, and learning potential, as well as the effectiveness of current research in that area.

Site Plan

Who are the nation's military and veteran caregivers? Existing published studies, including RAND's own, describe the unique attributes of the nation's military and veteran caregivers, highlighting the important ways in which they differ from the broader population of caregivers in the United States. However, stakeholder participants pointed to gaps in the existing knowledge about certain groups of military and veteran caregivers, as well as caregivers more broadly—for example, children, caregivers for whom English is not a first language, male caregivers, caregivers with preexisting or chronic medical conditions, college-aged caregivers, caregivers with disabled children, and caregivers of those who served in the military before the terrorist attacks of September 11, 2001 (9/11). While this objective was not rated as very important or of high learning potential among our stakeholders, it is likely that, as the needs of care recipients change, demographic trends shift, and the landscape of care for families continues to transform, describing caregivers will become increasingly important.

What societal cost savings can be attributed to caregivers? Caregivers play a critical role in supporting the needs of their care recipients, often enabling them to live in noninstitutionalized settings. The reliance on informal caregivers often defrays costs associated with formal caregiving. Smaller families, an increasingly aging population, and growing participation of women in the workforce are among the trends that will change not only who assumes the role of a caregiver but also the landscape of cost savings attributed to caregiving. Our stakeholder participants rated this objective as very important, noting that it should also include the expenses that military and veteran caregivers must bear; in other words, the research should include the trade-offs of caregiving. Stakeholder participants noted that caregivers themselves do not stand to benefit in their daily lives from research on this objective. However, understanding who military and veteran caregivers are and the benefits they convey to society can help guide programs and policies for caregivers that would lead to a more direct effect.

Floor Plan

How does caregiving affect caregivers? While several studies have documented the short-term impact of caregiving for those supporting individuals with specific age-related health conditions (such as dementia), little is known about the longer-term impact of caregiving on military and veteran caregivers in particular. Some stakeholder participants felt more was known about this topic than about other issues. However, they noted that understanding how caregiving affects caregivers could help inform programs and policies designed to mitigate any adverse effects. In addition, caregivers felt that research could help them "tell their story," noting that more public education and public awareness are needed.

Many panelists mentioned the importance of focusing on health, employment, and family well-being outcomes. Health, especially mental health, was prominently highlighted. Employment issues meant loss of income for some; for others, it meant the loss of a job opportunity or having to leave a much-valued position. Issues related to family functioning included family strain, divorce, and abuse.

One caregiver commented that there were also good consequences of caregiving, reminding us that studies should include the full range of caregiving effects, both positive and negative.

How does caregiving affect the children of caregivers? We could find no published studies about how caregiving affects a caregiver's children, but all of our stakeholder participants, particularly those in the caregiver panel, felt it was a vital topic, making this a high priority for future research. Panelists felt that the issue had the following aspects that merited attention: children directly serving as caregivers, the impact of being a child in a home with someone (usually a parent) caring for an individual with a mental health issue, the impact of caregiving on parenting and the associated effect on children, and both short-term and long-term effects of caregiving on children.

Children were viewed by many as "the forgotten secondary caregivers." Caregivers raised the topic of how children are affected by living in homes in which caregivers (usually their parents) are caring for someone with a mental health condition. Discussion of this topic often overlapped with the effects of caregiver parenting. Here, issues included a child competing for attention and the parent not meeting societal expectations, such as attending outings or field trips.

Over the short term, the effects of being the child of a caregiver were reflected in school performance, attachment issues, socialization, adverse behavior, and mental health. Panelists were not specific about the long-term outcomes of greatest interest, but the need for longitudinal research was highlighted, especially by program leaders, even while acknowledging that such research would be costly.

There was no agreement among stakeholders about whether it would be culturally acceptable to conduct research on the impact of caregiving on children. While some found the research objective too important to overlook, others thought that some parents might be unwilling to share insights about their children for fear of being criticized.

How does caregiving affect care recipients? Caregivers play an essential role in supporting the recovery and reintegration of our wounded, ill, and injured veterans by helping coordinate medical care, administer medications, and provide supportive environments. Some research has been done to examine the impact of caregiving on care recipient outcomes. However, the majority of that research has focused on short-term outcomes, and there is a limited understanding of the long-term outcomes; therefore, more studies are needed, particularly for military and veteran caregiving. ExpertLens participants saw this question as critical for justifying continued support for programs and services for caregivers. One panel member noted, "We need to be able to show [the benefit of caregiving for care recipient outcomes] to make the case for continued and increased funding." Furthermore, program leaders commented, "This would be useful in designing programs for support"; and "If resources are to be increased that are targeted to caregivers, there must be strong evidence of need and impact." One leader summed it up as follows: "We are in an outcomes-driven world. Documenting the outcomes is critical."

Some program leaders felt that much is already known about this topic, but they observed that much can be learned about how to improve the mental health and quality of life of military families. In particular, they saw the "journey" of post-9/11 veterans and their caregivers as a valuable source of baseline knowledge. The need for longitudinal research was again highlighted. Some program leaders felt that this topic might be sensitive because of the potential perceptions associated with caregiving (e.g., that caregivers may have lower productivity in the workplace) and needing or receiving care.

How do care recipient needs change over time? As individuals age or recover, their needs and demands for caregiving may change, and this may affect the duties and strain on the caregiver. However, only two studies published to date have examined how care recipients' needs change over time. This topic was widely viewed as extremely important among our stakeholders; research in this area could, for example, ensure that caregiver skills and knowledge keep pace with the changes in care recipient needs over time. Several program leaders felt that the focus should be on the long-term needs of different populations because "these needs might vary greatly by type of injury, type of care, and myriad other factors." Along these lines, one caregiver thought that society is more accepting of a Vietnam-era veteran needing care than a post-9/11 veteran, which is likely tied to a perception that older individuals require such support. The idea of a veteran in his or her 20s or 30s needing a caregiver seemed overwhelming and potentially expensive in the long run, but given the age of most post-9/11 veterans, more research on this topic is needed.

What factors are associated with caregiver and care recipient harm (that is, any situation in which a care recipient is abusing the caregiver or vice versa)? Fraud, harm, and abuse are often unpopular topics of discussion, but research with civilian populations indicates that this area deserves serious attention. Understanding the extent to which these issues occur and why they occur is important for safeguarding caregivers and care recipients and minimizing adverse consequences. But the effort is complicated by the stigma associated with admitting that a caregiver or care recipient is abusive in some way. Program leaders thought that getting honest answers about abuse would be prohibitively difficult but that people would likely self-report if they felt something good would result and the information was confidential. One leader summed up the potential for work in this area by noting that "we can actually make a huge difference in five years by adding this research goal into the mix." However, because of the sensitive nature of this topic, some felt that original, potentially expensive studies would be needed.

Caregivers and program leaders did not agree about whether to study medical fraud among caregivers and recipients. As an example of potential fraud, some noted that because a family could lose medical benefits and payments when a care recipient's health improves, that could be a disincentive for improved health. Stakeholders also acknowledged that it is very disruptive to a family to take away the stipend of a care recipient if his or her health improves. Losing benefits was a frightening prospect for caregivers, although all caregivers said that what they wanted most was for the health of their care recipient to improve. Thus, to ensure a full understanding of the risks and consequences associated with these issues, further research is necessary.

Elevation
What are strategies for making effective programs more accessible to more caregivers? Few studies have focused on the accessibility of caregiver programs that provide training, peer support, or health services, and no research has been done to understand the efficacy or effectiveness of workplace policies to support caregivers. Program leaders suggested that social media would be the most effective way to reach caregivers. Caregivers suggested a broader range of ways to learn about programs, including social media, word of mouth, sporting events, retreats, peer support networks, and Internet searches, among others. Furthermore, caregivers noted that a program might be accessible but not always available (e.g., there is a waiting list). They also expressed concerns

that caregivers might be reluctant to use such programs because doing so may suggest that the caregiver could not handle his or her responsibilities. However, there was general agreement that this was an important topic for future research.

How effective are programs and policies for ensuring caregiver well-being? Knowing what works and for whom is an important consideration not only for ensuring that caregivers' needs are being met but also for developing sound policies and funding worthy efforts. Many programs and policies have been promulgated in health care settings, in the workplace, and in the social support arena with the intent of improving caregiver well-being.

Very little of the existing research focused on proving the efficacy of specific caregiver interventions. Instead, the vast majority of research was on the effectiveness of programs enhancing caregivers' abilities to provide care, including informal and formal education and training, assessments of caregiver knowledge and information programs, and programs using new technologies (e.g., telehealth, smartphones) to help caregivers with caregiving tasks. About one-third of the literature on program effectiveness focused on care recipients with dementia.

How effective are programs and policies for supporting caregivers' ability to provide care? Although this question has been fairly well studied in the past, caregivers felt that they did not have the information they needed to provide required care and were unaware of research on the effectiveness of key programs. They also criticized the ongoing, exhausting, and often disorganized bureaucratic aspects of programs and policies.

Considering Cross-Cutting Issues

Some issues cut across the research blueprint. Many stemmed from the lack of studies on specific subpopulations of caregivers, especially children and men. Research on these populations should consider how caregiving affects them in ways that may be unique or different from the impact experienced by adults (in the case of children) and by women or spouses (in the case of men, some of whom may be providing care for friends). Studies should also specifically address the efficacy and effectiveness of programs or policies for these groups.

A second cross-cutting concern was the lack of research focused on those caring for a particular type of care recipient—for example, those with a brain injury. A large longitudinal study currently being conducted by the U.S. Department of Defense to examine the caregivers of service members who experienced a traumatic brain injury during the post-9/11 era will provide valuable insights, but additional research will be needed to ensure that all health issues affecting caregivers are studied.

Using the Blueprint

Ideally, the research blueprint we have created will become a common reference point for the various stakeholder communities as they work toward a common goal of improving support for military and veteran caregivers. We suggest the following three strategies for gaining support for, adopting, and implementing the blueprint.

Establish partnerships. The military and veteran caregiver stakeholder community can partner with some of the many organizations that are interested in research on various aspects of caregiving. For example, the National Academies of Science, Engineering, and Medicine's Committee on Family Caregiving for Older Adults released a report in September 2016 outlining recommendations aimed at addressing the health, economic, and social issues facing family caregivers of older Americans; many of the recommendations are also relevant to military and veteran caregivers because many of their care recipients are elderly (National Academies of Science, Engineering, and Medicine, 2016).

Among other recommendations, the committee suggested that the U.S. Department of Veterans Affairs and the U.S. Department of Health and Human Services create a public-private, multistakeholder fund for research and innovation to accelerate the pace of change in addressing the needs of caregiving families. The research objectives that we evaluated and arrayed within this blueprint can all be nested within these larger objectives and used as a basis for informing how the Department of Veterans Affairs and Department of Defense in particular can support and implement this recommendation.

Additional partnerships and consortia with other caregiver organizations could be established to call for increased research investment, encourage the research community to focus on caregiving, and demand more evidence-based decisionmaking for future caregiver support programs and policies.

Convene a military and veteran caregiver research summit. A research summit could be convened to focus on cultivating new research studies designed around elements identified in this research blueprint. Participants could include researchers from multiple disciplines, as well as caregiver representatives.

Create a research center of excellence. A research center of excellence within the military and veteran caregiving community could foster the strategic pursuit of the research blueprint and begin to address the knowledge gaps outlined in this report, thus promoting better support for military and veteran caregivers in the future.

Acknowledgments

We are grateful to many organizations and individuals who contributed to this analysis and report. This study was made possible thanks to the Elizabeth Dole Foundation, a nonprofit organization dedicated to advancing solutions to address the challenges and long-term needs that military caregivers face. We thank Senator Elizabeth Dole and Steve Schwab at the Foundation for their leadership. We thank our technical peer reviewers, James F. Malec and Thomas Concannon, for their constructive feedback on the report; Quiana Fulton for her administrative assistance on the project; and Mary Vaiana for her help in improving the report. Finally, we thank the many military and veteran caregivers, fellow researchers, caregiver advocates, and caregiver support program leaders who took the time to fill out surveys, share their ideas, and/or participate in the ExpertLens process.

CHAPTER ONE

Introduction

There are more than 20 million veterans living in the United States today, a significant portion of whom have service-connected conditions or disabilities that require ongoing support and care. Supporting these wounded, ill, and injured warriors are the nation's "hidden heroes"—caregivers who provide unpaid, informal support with activities that enable current and former U.S. service members to live fuller lives and who are an essential component of the nation's care for returning warriors. Recently, these caregivers have been the subject of much national attention. Starting in 2010, new federal programs were created to ensure improved support for caregivers; however, at the time, little was known about the characteristics and needs of this population.

In 2014, the RAND Corporation published *Hidden Heroes: America's Military Caregivers*, which shed light on the number and characteristics of these military and veteran caregivers and the burden they face in providing informal care and support to current and former U.S. service members (Ramchand, Tanielian, et al., 2014).[1] The study was the first to rigorously describe the population of these caregivers, the value they contribute to society, and the risks they face as a result of their caregiving roles. The RAND study also canvassed the existing programs and policies that support military and veteran caregivers and highlighted gaps in that support landscape.

Four of the study findings were of particular importance and serve as context for this report. First, of the 5.5 million individuals who were providing care and assistance to a current or former member of the U.S. armed forces, 20 percent (1.1 million) were supporting an individual who served in the era after the terrorist attacks of September 11, 2001 (9/11). Second, the study found important demographic, health, and labor force participation differences between caregivers of those who served before 9/11 and of those who served after. Third, it found that, while there were many programs designed to support caregivers, there were gaps in access for some caregivers of post-9/11 service members (based on age, relationship to, or condition of the care recipient).

---

[1] We use the term *military and veteran caregiver* to be inclusive of both those caring for a current member of the military (including active-duty, reserve, and National Guard members) and those caring for a former member of the military (commonly referred to as a veteran).

Fourth, the study identified significant threats to the future of military caregiving—based, most notably, on the aging of the population and the increasing stress faced by young spouses.

Given the important contribution that caregivers make in ensuring the recovery and reintegration of U.S. service members and veterans, the 2014 RAND report also outlined recommendations for ensuring better support for military and veteran caregivers in the future. Among these recommendations was a call for increased investment in research on the population. The recommendation had the following three components:

- Ensure continued research into the evolving need for caregiving assistance among U.S. service members and veterans, particularly for post-9/11 service members as they age, and the resulting evolving demands on their caregivers.
- Conduct additional and continued research to document the needs of and outcomes for caregivers so that interventions can be better tailored or targeted to reduce or mitigate the negative consequences associated with caregiving.
- Increase the amount of research that identifies the efficacy (i.e., whether an intervention has the intended effect under ideal circumstances) and effectiveness (i.e., whether an intervention has the intended effect in usual, real-world conditions) of caregiver support programs and policies to ensure that resources are being used efficiently and that evidence-based programs and policies are promulgated. Where programs and policies have not been rigorously assessed according to evidence-based practice criteria, they should nevertheless be rooted in relevant outcome data and the best available research from peer-reviewed publications.

Since the release of the 2014 study, there has been action on many of the recommendations, including additional research funding to evaluate specific military and veteran caregiver support programs. For example, the U.S. Department of Veterans Affairs (VA) launched an evaluation of its Comprehensive Caregiver Support Program, and the Bristol Myers Squibb Foundation funded an evaluation of the Military Veteran Caregiver Network. While these studies will yield valuable insights on whether specific programs have been effective, longitudinal research is still needed to inform our understanding of how caregiver needs evolve over time as caregivers age and their care recipients' needs change, how specific programs are working, and how caregiving affects specific subgroups of caregivers. In response to these needs, the Elizabeth Dole Foundation requested that RAND develop a *research blueprint* to guide future investments in this area.

The Role of a Blueprint

Blueprints have been developed to guide research across health conditions (e.g., child and adolescent mental health: Hoagwood and Olin, 2002; pediatric oncology: Park et al., 2013). However, there is no consensus on what a research blueprint entails. To guide our project, we turned to the field from which the term *blueprint* originates: architecture and construction. Before a new house is constructed, an architect investigates where it will be built, talks with the owners about what their needs will be, and investigates the laws and regulations that guide what can be designed. The architect then creates a design for the new house and displays it in a blueprint that communicates the design intent to both the owners and the builder. The blueprint also functions as the contract among these parties, documenting and specifying the decisions about what is to be constructed.

A blueprint for caregiving research can be considered in the same way. With support from the Elizabeth Dole Foundation, input from key stakeholders, and a review of caregiving research to date, RAND researchers serve as the architects, conveying a vision for research needed to "build the house" (in this case, ensure better support for military and veteran caregivers). Members of the research community, who will be responsible for executing the research, serve as the builders. Note that a construction blueprint is not a manual for erecting a building; rather, it merely communicates the architect's design intent, and it is the builder's responsibility to acquire the means and methods with which to execute that intent. Similarly, in this blueprint for caregiving research, we do not specify *how* researchers should go about addressing specific research questions; rather, we describe the research questions that should be prioritized. Allowing builders creative license in interpreting an architect's design can result in economic efficiencies, technological advances, and new insights, and we believe that giving researchers the same creative license can yield the same results.

The owner of the research—that is, who will ultimately live in and benefit from the house—is the public, including caregivers and care recipients, as well as those who support them. An architect should design a building with the owners' needs at the forefront of her mind, not her own interests or those of the builder. In designing this blueprint, we pursued a similar goal: to keep caregivers, care recipients, and those who support them in the forefront of our minds, prioritizing research that will best serve their needs.

In addition to the architects, builders, and owners in this blueprint metaphor, we can think of program leaders as the suppliers, who ensure that the house is built with the best available materials, and we can think of policymakers as the inspectors, who ensure that it has been examined and approved.

Components of a Blueprint

In architecture, a blueprint has many components, but three are primary: site plan, floor plan, and elevation.

A *site plan* shows the footprint of a building on a given lot, including the pathways connecting the structure to the lot (e.g., sidewalks, pipes). In caregiving research, an analogous construct is *research that examines how caregiving and caregivers fit within the context of society at large.* Such research quantifies how many caregivers there are and describes who they are and for whom they provide care. It may also quantify social benefits associated with caregiving—for example, by estimating societal cost savings attributed to unpaid, informal caregiving.

A *floor plan* describes the relationships between rooms and spaces on one floor within the building and how to move between them (e.g., interior doors, hallways). In caregiving research, an analogous construct is *research that examines how caregiving affects caregivers.* For example, it may include studies that assess how caregiver demands change as the needs of those they are caring for change, as well as how caregiving affects caregivers, care recipients, and caregivers' families (including their children). It may also examine factors associated with caregiver and care recipient harm (for example, any situation in which a care recipient is abusing the caregiver or vice versa).

An *elevation* shows the building from the outside, providing a view of the exterior doors and windows that allow people inside the house to look out or exit and that allow people outside to look in or enter. In caregiving research, an analogous construct is *research that examines how external factors may influence the caregiving experience.* For example, such research may identify strategies for supporting caregivers through new policies or programs, making current programs more available to caregivers, or evaluating the effectiveness of policies or programs.

Site plans, floor plans, and elevations are all necessary to ensure that builders have the perspectives and information necessary to construct a house. One plan is not given priority over the other, but each of the plans reveals the details that may make the house more stable or may make living in it more enjoyable. Other details may be exceedingly difficult for builders to construct but are important to include nonetheless. In adopting the blueprint analogy, we similarly do not prioritize research ideas; rather, we describe how some research priorities may better support the well-being of caregivers over the long term, and others may be exceedingly difficult for researchers to address but are important to pursue.

Organization of This Report

The remainder of this report is organized into three sections. In Chapter Two, we describe our methods and resources in building the research blueprint. In Chapter Three, we describe the components of the blueprint, outlining the necessary conditions for enabling the blueprint's execution and sketching out the site plan, floor plan, and elevation. Chapter Four describes how to use the blueprint and provides recommendations for how to move forward with implementation. Additional methodological details are included in the electronic appendixes to this report.

CHAPTER TWO
Methods

Because creating an architectural blueprint requires a variety of technical expertise, the RAND team sought to gather multiple forms of data and garner insights from those who know the field best. We used input from the following five sources:

- observation and documentation of conference sessions at the "Empowering Hidden Heroes: Pathways to InnoVAtion" summit, cosponsored by the Elizabeth Dole Foundation and the VA
- a free-listing exercise among attendees at the summit
- a survey administered to attendees at the summit
- a research inventory through a review of the literature
- stakeholder consensus evaluation using ExpertLens™—a RAND-developed, web-based tool that assesses stakeholder consensus.

We submitted the protocol for this study to RAND's Human Subjects Protection Committee for review, and the committee deemed it exempt.

Data Collection at the "Empowering Hidden Heroes: Pathways to InnoVAtion" Summit

In September 2016, our four-person study team attended the "Empowering Hidden Heroes: Pathways to InnoVAtion" summit. This seminal, one-day event in Washington, D.C., brought together 267 stakeholders, including policy and program officials, government officials, researchers, clinicians, funders, advocates, care recipients, and caregivers.

Observation and Documentation of Panels and Attendee Reactions at the Summit
During the event, we attended eight individual and panel presentations and spoke with summit attendees to elicit their general perspectives on future research to support military and veteran caregivers. Each team member took notes throughout, paying particular attention to recurring themes, key questions raised by attendees, mention

of future directions in caregiver research and advocacy, and attendee reactions to the issues addressed. As observers at the event, we were able to familiarize ourselves with the current state of caregiver advocacy and research, strengthen rapport, conduct unstructured interviews with attendees, and recruit stakeholders to inform the development of this blueprint. Our notes served as a foundation for framing the review of data collected during the free-listing exercise described next.

Free-Listing Exercise

We conducted a free-listing exercise in which attendees were invited to anonymously write on an index card which research priorities for caregivers they perceived as the most pressing, relevant, or useful to pursue and then post the cards to a board for others to read. We set up a table next to the board where we provided information on this blueprint study, engaged attendees in conversation, and recorded notes on our interactions with attendees. As the board became populated with research priorities, we used it to elicit feedback and personal experiences with caregiving (i.e., an elicitation technique).

After the summit, we compiled our notes (e.g., "a male caregiver mentioned that he feels that male caregivers go under-recognized in the caregiving community") and pooled them into a list. Drawing on our expertise in the topic (our team was led by experts on military and veteran caregiving) and qualitative data analysis, we identified the following research domains:

- the caregiving population, including subgroups (e.g., male caregivers)
- types of interventions needed for caregivers (e.g., promoting the healthy involvement of children in caregiving)
- clinical conditions of care recipients (e.g., care recipients with traumatic brain injury)
- social impacts of caregiving (e.g., emotional and mental health impacts of caregiving)
- cross-cutting themes (e.g., financial impact of caregiving, impact of caregiving on children).

We then sorted each of the free-listing index cards into one of these research domains. We combined these topics with the existing research topics identified in RAND's previous research on military and veteran caregivers. We then triangulated these research topics with the findings from a survey conducted at the summit, described next.

Survey

Our third form of data collection at the summit was a survey (see Appendix A) designed to assess levels of support for and prioritization of potential research objectives on the well-being of caregivers. This comprehensive list of objectives was developed from RAND's existing research on military and veteran caregivers and expert knowledge from the project leads prior to the conference as a means to gather feedback on some general areas of research. The survey asked respondents to use Likert scales to *rate the importance of research* on

- types of caregivers (e.g., children, parents, men)
- positive and negative consequences of caregiving (e.g., health-related problems)
- conditions and disabilities of care recipients (e.g., brain injury, posttraumatic stress disorder)
- efforts and programs for caregivers.

The survey also asked respondents to *rate overall strategies* for understanding and evaluating caregiver well-being and caregiver programs. These strategies included

- understanding the needs of the caregiver population
- understanding the needs of the care recipient population
- documenting or assessing the positive and negative impacts of caregiving
- examining unique aspects associated with specific conditions
- assessing the efficacy or effectiveness of programs
- evaluating policies
- other (respondents were asked to specify).

The survey concluded with an open-ended response on *where research on caregiving is most needed*. Our purpose in including this wide array of questions and topics, as well as the open-ended response, was to ensure that all potential research objectives were considered prior to our ExpertLens rating exercise (described later).

We disseminated the survey to all participants at the summit, and we received 158 completed surveys (a 59-percent response rate). The written survey took respondents 15 minutes to complete, on average.

After compiling data gathered at the summit, we identified 16 potential research objectives for studying caregivers (see Appendix B). These were intended to be umbrella objectives that could cover the breadth and depth of topics and needs expressed by participants at the summit. As will be explained later, we ultimately shortened the list of 16 objectives to ten.

Research Inventory

The aim of the research inventory was to conduct a scan of the literature to identify the existing evidence base (i.e., where evidence is robust or scant) for supporting military and veteran caregivers. We used the 16 research objectives we identified (see Appendix B) as an organizing framework for assessing how the identified literature could be distributed across the different areas of interest. To achieve a full scan of the existing evidence base for supporting military and veteran caregivers, we broadened our research to include literature on multiple types of caregivers (e.g., for the elderly).

We searched electronic databases (PsychINFO, Social Science Abstracts, PubMed, and PILOTS-Pro Quest) to identify all published articles, books, reports, and book reviews on caregiving issues among military, veteran, and civilian populations between 2005 and 2017. We included all empirical, descriptive, or experimental studies that described an adult disability or condition and a caregiver. We excluded all studies that involved caregiving for children, did not mention caregivers or an adult disability or condition, or were performed outside the United States.

One member of our study team verified the abstracts and sources for the publications. Because the aim was to assess the evidence base and not summarize detailed research findings, we did not conduct a systematic full-text review. We used the title and abstract to code publications for the following key variables: author, title, year published, type of publication, journal title or publisher name, and disabilities or conditions mentioned.

We also coded the "study goal" of the publication into one of the 16 research objectives. In a spreadsheet, one researcher coded for the presence (or absence) of a category as a binary variable (0 or 1), stratified by the type of publication (e.g., book chapter, journal article). The presence or absence of literature in these areas, based on the actual counts of publications, depicts where the evidence base is robust and where it is weak—that is, where more research may be needed. See Appendix C.

ExpertLens

Once we identified the 16 research objectives, we sought to better understand how stakeholders rated them with respect to the following five dimensions:

1. *importance* of the research objective (we asked, how important overall is pursuing this research objective for improving support for military and veteran caregivers?)
2. *effectiveness* of previous research in the area (we asked, how effective have studies pursuing this research objective been for supporting military and veteran caregivers in the past?)
3. *cultural acceptability* of conducting the research (we asked, how culturally acceptable are research studies that pursue this research objective?)
4. *implementation cost* of performing the research (we asked, how expensive do you believe it is to conduct studies focused on this research objective?)

5. the *learning potential* of the research in the next five years (we asked, how much could we learn in the next five years by funding research pursuant to this goal?).

These dimensions were drawn from a prior objective-rating exercise employed among a varied stakeholder community for designing a research strategy in suicide prevention (Claassen et al., 2014). Similar criteria, including cultural appropriateness, feasibility, and importance, have also been tested and validated in other studies (see Khodyakov et al., 2016). To collect data in an efficient and standardized way, we used the RAND-developed system ExpertLens, which uses a three-step, web-based elicitation process to gather input from stakeholders. ExpertLens combines both qualitative and quantitative approaches to systematically and iteratively gather input and gauge consensus on complex issues. It has been used in more than a dozen studies among a wide range of stakeholder groups, including researchers, program leaders, funders, community members, and advocates, and on topics as diverse as suicide prevention (Ramchand, Eberhart, et al., 2014) and ethics in translational science (Khodyakov et al., 2016).

During an initial, internal pilot of the ExpertLens panel, we learned that respondents felt that 16 research objectives were too many to report on and that there was enough overlap among certain priorities to warrant a shorter list. Thus, before implementing the ExpertLens process, we condensed the number of research objectives to ten. The shorter list streamlined the selection of research objectives and made the list more manageable for study participants. The final ten objectives are as follows (see Appendix B for the original 16 objectives):

1. Assess how the needs of care recipients (e.g., assistance with activities of daily living, instrumental activities of daily living, level of disability) change over time.
2. Quantify the societal cost savings attributed to caregiving.
3. Assess the consequences of caregiving on the children of caregivers.
4. Identify strategies for making effective programs available to more caregivers.
5. Describe caregivers (e.g., identify characteristics of those who provide care, how many serve in this role).
6. Evaluate the effectiveness of programs and policies for ensuring caregiver well-being (e.g., evaluate respite services, workplace flexibility).
7. Document the effects of caregiving on care recipient outcomes (e.g., health, well-being, need for assistance).
8. Document the effects of caregiving on caregiver outcomes (e.g., fatigue, divorce, disruption to work or school schedules, disruption to childcare, mental and physical health).
9. Examine factors associated with caregiver and care recipient harm (e.g., abuse, medical fraud).

10. Identify effective programs and policies (e.g., training, health care policies, workplace policies) to support caregivers' ability to provide care.

Recruitment

We used a purposeful sampling approach to populate three kinds of panels based on stakeholder type: caregivers; researchers, government and policy officials, and funders (RGF); and program leaders. The study team initiated recruitment at the "Empowering Hidden Heroes: Pathways to InnoVAtion" summit, where we informed the diverse group of attendees about the ExpertLens panels and provided a website where participants could register. In addition, we emailed additional researchers and program leaders working on military and veteran caregiver issues to invite them to participate in an ExpertLens panel. Lastly, the Elizabeth Dole Foundation assisted with recruitment by posting a link to the panels on Twitter and encouraging followers to register.

A total of 263 stakeholders registered online to participate in an ExpertLens panel. To keep the sizes of our three panel types roughly equivalent, we randomized the 180 caregivers into four panels of roughly 45. The RGF panel included 39 participants, and the final panel included 44 program leaders. Each stakeholder was advised that participation entailed three rounds (see next subsection). To qualify as a respondent, the stakeholder had to log in, register, and participate in the rating exercise during either round one or round three (participants in round two were encouraged but not required). See Appendix B for additional information about the characteristics of the ExpertLens panelists.

Data Collection

Each panel completed a three-round web-based ExpertLens process throughout November 2016. In round one, participants rated each of the ten research objectives with respect to the five dimensions (importance, effectiveness, cultural acceptability, implementation cost, and learning potential) on a 9-point Likert scale format. Participants were requested, but not required, to provide a rationale for their response in text boxes. The order of the research objectives was randomized to reduce participant bias.

In round two, participants were shown how their round-one ratings and rationales compared with those from other panelists in their groups. Panelists then engaged in anonymous, asynchronous, electronic discussions regarding the evaluation criteria and other comments from a general discussion board. We monitored and moderated these discussions at multiple points to clarify rationale and stimulate discussion. Participants could provide rationale either for a particular criterion directly or to a general discussion board for each of the ten research objectives.

In round three, we showed panelists the same format as in round one and asked them to reevaluate the research objectives, taking into account the information they had been exposed to in round two. We then calculated a final rating for each dimension under each research objective, stratified across panels. As before, the order of the research objectives was randomized to reduce participant bias.

Completion of all three rounds differed across the panels (see Table 2.1). Because participation in ExpertLens is anonymous, there is no way to determine whether non-respondents differed from respondents in significant ways. It is also not possible to know why panelists rated some criteria but not others (e.g., we do not know whether a user simply committed an error or was uninterested in the criteria). We combined the data from the four caregiver panels, but because we wanted to preserve the different perspectives of the stakeholder types, we did not combine any other panels.

Data Analysis

Our research plan is shown in Figure 2.1. As described earlier, we used data collected at the "Empowering Hidden Heroes: Pathways to InnoVAtion" summit to identify the initial 16 research objectives. We achieved this through triangulation of the categories identified through RAND's existing research; through the free-listing exercise, discussions, and observations at the summit; and through the ratings and rankings in the survey. These objectives were used to structure a literature review, and we coded the study goal of each publication into one of our 16 research objectives. The literature review systematically identified the evidence base for these objectives, outlining where existing research could be used to inform a research objective, as well as where more research is needed to address the needs of military and veteran caregivers.

Table 2.1
ExpertLens Participation

	Round 1 (Those Who Rated More Than Half the Dimensions)	Round 2 (Those Who Posted to a Discussion)	Round 3 (Those Who Participated in Round One and Rated More Than Half the Dimensions in Round Three)
Caregiver panel 1	22.7% (10/44)	13.6% (6/44)	23.5% (4/17)
Caregiver panel 2	21.7% (10/46)	4.3% (2/46)	14.3% (2/14)
Caregiver panel 3	22.2% (10/45)	17.8% (8/45)	18.8% (3/16)
Caregiver panel 4	35.6% (16/45)	22.2% (10/45)	22.7% (5/22)
RGF panel	17.9% (7/39)	10.3% (4/39)	30.0% (3/10)
Program leader panel	31.8% (14/44)	18.2% (8/44)	29.4% (5/17)

NOTE: The denominator values reflect the total number of participants who logged into their respective panel, and the numerator values show the number of participants who both logged in to participate and provided ratings for more than half of the objectives and their related evaluation criteria.

Figure 2.1
Analytic Strategy

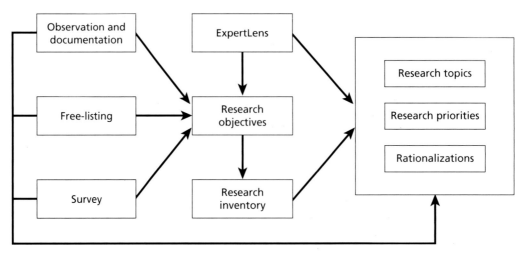

Through iterative feedback among the study team, as well as an internal pilot test of ExpertLens, we identified objectives that were similar in their scope. For example, we subsumed "Evaluate the effectiveness of *workplace policies* (e.g., flexible work schedules, support lines) in supporting caregivers" and "Evaluate the effectiveness of *health care policies* (e.g., revisions to privacy laws, changes to screening procedures) in supporting caregivers" into "Evaluate the effectiveness of programs and policies for ensuring caregiver well-being (e.g., evaluate respite services, workplace flexibility)." This led us to condense the initial list of 16 research objectives to ten. Via ExpertLens, we asked stakeholders to rate and comment on these objectives across five dimensions (importance, effectiveness, cultural acceptability, implementation cost, and learning potential). Primarily from these sources, we were able to identify specific research topics within each objective, as well as rationales for studying such topics. This information was then exported from ExpertLens into tables showing the median rating of the five dimensions for each of the three panel types (caregivers, RGF, and program leaders).

Panel results from ExpertLens were determined using the process described in the *RAND/UCLA Appropriateness Method User's Manual* (Fitch et al., 2001; see also Khodyakov et al., 2016). We report the ExpertLens categorization of ratings, which automatically translates the median from the 9-point numerical rating system into a categorical rating (e.g., uncertain, important, unimportant, acceptable, unacceptable, effective, ineffective, high, low). Median panel ratings between 1 and 3 were rated as unimportant, ineffective, unacceptable, high implementation cost, or low learning potential (depending on the dimension), while panel ratings between 7 and 9 were rated as important, effective, acceptable, low implementation cost, or high learning potential. Uncertainty was classified in two ways: when the median fell between 4 and

6 on the 9-point scale for a given dimension or when there was disagreement within the panel. Disagreement occurred when more than one-third of the participants chose a rating between 1 and 3 and more than one-third chose a rating between 7 and 9. Throughout this report, we note when the three panels rated dimensions for particular objectives differently (e.g., for the research objective to describe caregivers, the importance dimension was rated by caregivers and the RGF panel to be important, but program leaders rated it as uncertain).

To determine the range of perspectives on each of the research objectives, we first triangulated the ratings with the rationales and comments across the dimensions, objectives, and panels. In particular, we examined the discussion comments and rationales for agreement and disagreement with the overall panel rating. Hence, we used a two-step process in which we drew on the qualitative data, such as respondent comments in round two, to inform *why* panel participants rated the objectives as they did. This elicited the thought processes behind each rating, offered details on the range of responses, provided quotations to illustrate overall stakeholder support for each priority, and demonstrated how participants drew links among the objectives.

We next sought to reach consensus on how each of the ten research objectives aligned with the purpose of the *site plan*, *floor plan*, and *elevation* of the blueprint described in Chapter One. While we agreed that the objectives are interrelated, we found that grouping them as shown in Table 2.2 was useful for outlining future research to improve support for caregivers.

Table 2.2
Research Objectives and Organization of the Blueprint

Blueprint Component	Focus	Research Objectives
Site plan	Caregivers as members of society	• Describe caregivers. • Quantify the societal cost savings attributed to caregiving.
Floor plan	Impacts of caregiving on caregivers, care recipients, and their families	• Document the effects of caregiving on caregiver outcomes. • Assess the consequences of caregiving on the children of caregivers. • Document the effects of caregiving on care recipient outcomes. • Assess how the needs of care recipients change over time. • Examine factors associated with caregiver and care recipient harm.
Elevation	External factors that influence caregiving	• Identify strategies for making effective programs available to more caregivers. • Evaluate the effectiveness of programs and policies for ensuring caregiver well-being. • Identify effective programs and policies to support caregivers' ability to provide care.

CHAPTER THREE

The Blueprint

Getting Started: Understanding Necessary Conditions

Having a blueprint is not sufficient for constructing a building; many other requirements must also be met. These can include acquiring the necessary building permits, hiring the appropriate personnel, and allotting the necessary financial resources. Similarly, to implement a research blueprint, multiple conditions must be met. We outline a few here as the starting point for readying the field and the community to implement the research blueprint described in this chapter. But many other critical steps also must be met in implementing the research. These may include, among others, scientific and ethical review for specific study proposals and, depending on the funder or the type of research, stakeholder involvement plans and pilot data.

Terminology, Definitions, and Measures

Within the field of informal caregiving, stakeholders may define the population or the tasks associated with caregiving differently. These definitions can lead to different inclusion and exclusion criteria for studies. For purposes of this blueprint, we define a *military and veteran caregiver* as anyone who provides unpaid care and assistance for, or manages the care of, a current or former member of the U.S. military, National Guard, or reserves who has an illness, injury, or condition for which they require outside support. Our definition is not limited to a familial relationship with the care recipient or to assistance provided for specific activities of daily living.

In addition to specifying the population of interest for a research blueprint, it is essential to have well-defined outcomes of interest and to use accepted, validated measures. Although outcomes of interest may vary across stakeholder groups or types of researchers (e.g., economists may be more interested in financial outcomes or impacts related to workforce participation, whereas psychologists may be more interested in or inclined to measure outcomes focused on mental well-being, social isolation, or relationship burden), it is important that researchers conducting work on military and veteran caregivers be explicit in their definitions and use commonly accepted and well-validated measures of the constructs of interest. Doing so will enable more-rigorous comparison of studies and evaluation of program outcomes.

It is beyond the scope of this report to define all of the main constructs and outcomes that the field should pursue. Similarly, the blueprint does not establish common measures for the field; rather, it outlines a series of research objectives that if pursued will help create better support for military and veteran caregivers in the future.

Environment Conducive to Research

For additional research on military and veteran caregivers to proceed, other enablers will be necessary. These include ensuring an environment that is conducive to facilitating, conducting, and using research. We describe enablers of such an environment here.

Funding. Most researchers identify having dedicated research funding as a key enabler of their work. Funding can come from many sources across the public and private sectors. Most of the research to date on military and veteran caregivers has been funded by either the federal government (e.g., the VA and U.S. Department of Defense) or the nonprofit, philanthropic sector (e.g., the UnitedHealth Foundation, Elizabeth Dole Foundation, Bristol-Myers Squibb Foundation). However, other funders may be interested in and amenable to supporting research on military and veteran caregivers. Such funding will be necessary to ensure that sufficient resources are available to support rigorous research on the population.

Research workforce. Conducting research requires appropriately trained individuals to perform studies with rigor and to contribute their findings to the knowledge base. Many types of researchers, from multiple disciplines, will be needed to implement a research blueprint. Whether researchers are quantitatively or qualitatively focused, it is important that they use methods appropriate to the research objective and publish their findings so they are available to the research, advocacy, and decisionmaking communities. The process of technical peer review often helps to ensure the quality of the research and should be incorporated both at the time of funding or research implementation and at the publication or reporting phase. As more funding becomes available and research priorities are articulated, more researchers may be drawn to the field and help expand and strengthen the science.

Community participation. Ultimately, successfully implementing studies of military and veteran caregivers will require participation from relevant parties, whether it is caregivers or the programs or settings designed to support caregivers. Ensuring that the perspectives of these constituencies are appropriately considered and addressed in the design and conduct of research can be instrumental in facilitating successful implementation. Thus, mechanisms to formally engage members of the military and veteran caregiver stakeholder community in identifying research questions, implementing studies, and using research findings will be important to establish. This could happen at the individual-study level or, perhaps, at the portfolio-management level within a funding organization. An additional strategy would be to draw on Participatory Action Research, which is an established, mutually beneficial framework for systematically incorporating the views and needs of advocates and the communities of people they seek to help (McIntyre, 2007). Given the existing knowledge and zeal among Elizabeth Dole Foundation fellows, Participatory Action Research would be an effective means of leveraging advocates' strengths in future research efforts.

Vocal champions. The imperative to increase the knowledge base and research funding to support such studies can be generated and influenced by the affected community. Those who advocate better support for military and veteran caregivers can be important vocal champions in encouraging policymakers across the government and nongovernment sectors to increase their support for and reliance on research. This can include increases in research budgets, as well as increased demand for policymakers and program officials to require rigorous evidence to inform decisionmaking. Thus, policymakers are important champions and ambassadors for research. Making stakeholders and advocates an integral part of the research process, through such efforts as Participatory Action Research, increases the salience of the work and facilitates better dissemination and implementation of the findings.

Translating research into practice. Generating new knowledge will be key, but enhancing support for military and veteran caregivers will require translating findings into practice. Without specific dissemination or facilitation efforts, it can often take more than a decade for new findings to influence routine practice (Morris et al., 2011). It is possible to shorten this timeline, but it requires specific intention to do so. Past RAND research (Ramchand, Eberhart et al., 2014) has identified ten strategies that often promote the translation of research into practice; those strategies include creating incentives for implementing new findings in practice and using evaluation findings in decisionmaking. These tasks are typically outside the scope of individual researchers and may require stakeholder groups to take the lead in facilitating them.

Defined Research Objectives

Research is often conducted to answer specific questions, whether the questions are designed to generate purely descriptive information or to evaluate the impact of a new intervention or way of doing things. Defining the research question is an important first step in deciding how studies or evaluations should be conducted, what methods should be applied, and what analyses will be most appropriate for answering the question. Well-defined research questions or objectives may also serve to identify the most-appropriate potential funding sources and target audiences for sharing the findings. For example, the funders and policymakers interested in research designed to assess the impact of caregiving on the mental health of caregivers may be different from those interested in research designed to assess the impact of caregiving on the workforce productivity of caregivers. Similarly, focusing a question on a particular population, such as caregivers of those with a spinal disorder, might suggest different funding sources and dissemination opportunities.

Because there are many potential research questions and objectives that can inform how best to support military and veteran caregivers in the future, the research blueprint intends to offer a way to conceptualize and organize specific research objectives that various stakeholders identified as salient. The remainder of this chapter describes how the research objectives fit within the blueprint's site plan, floor plan, and elevation.

The Site Plan

We define the site plan of the caregiving research blueprint to include those research objectives that pertain to how the estimated 5.5 million military and veteran caregivers fit into the fabric of U.S. society. In this section, we explore research opportunities related to describing the range of attributes of military and veteran caregivers, as well as the societal cost savings that can be attributed to their efforts.

Describe Caregivers

A key aim of the 2014 RAND report *Hidden Heroes: America's Military Caregivers* was to describe the attributes of the 5.5 million (and growing) military and veteran caregivers in the United States. We know that individual caregivers have unique characteristics and strengths and that they differ widely in geographic region, age, employment status, race/ethnicity, and so on. More importantly, the 2014 report emphasized that the military and veteran caregiving population differs in notable ways from the broader population of caregivers in the United States. Our literature review identified 34 published works identifying characteristics and demographics of those who serve as caregivers (see Table 3.1). The majority of published works were journal articles focused on civilian populations; many of the sources also focused on the elderly, who present challenges to the caregiving enterprise that are different from those posed by military and veteran populations. This suggests that the evidence base on descriptions of caregivers can be considered fairly robust, albeit less so among the military and veteran caregiver populations.

However, as this section illustrates, less attention has been given to "minority" caregivers (e.g., male caregivers, caregivers for whom English is not a first language). Furthermore, describing caregivers is an ever-evolving task because the needs of care recipients change, demographic trends shift, and the landscape of care for our families continues to transform.

During our ExpertLens (stakeholder consensus evaluation) process, the caregiver and RGF panels rated the importance of research on describing caregivers (e.g., identifying characteristics of those who provide care, how many serve in this role) to be uncertain (median for caregiver panels = 6/9; for RGF panel = 6.5/9), while the program leader panel rated it to be of high importance (median = 7.5/9). However, all three panels were unsure about how much could be learned in the next five years by funding research that pursues this research objective (median for caregiver panels = 6/9; RGF panel = 6/9; program leader panel = 6.5/9). Hence, at present, stakeholders overall see

Table 3.1
Breakdown of Literature Examining Caregivers as Members of Society

	Number of Sources Describing Caregivers	Number of Sources Quantifying the Societal Cost Savings Attributed to Caregivers
Total	34	5
Type of publication		
Journal article	32	3
Book or report	2	2
Population		
Civilian	29	4
Military/veteran	5	1
Condition		
Dementia/Alzheimer's	8	2
Musculoskeletal injury	1	0
Heart disease	1	0
Stroke	1	0
Cancer	1	0
Brain injury	1	0
Paralysis	0	0
Burn	0	0
Mental illness	0	0
General elder care	4	2
Other	17	1

this objective as having uncertain importance and as less relevant or pressing than other less-studied research objectives. See Table 3.2 for all of the ratings, by dimension, for the research blueprint's site plan (that is, the research objectives on how caregivers fit into the broader society), including their categorization (e.g., uncertain, effective, high learning potential).

Overlooked Caregivers

Despite the lower priority ratings given to research on caregivers during the ExpertLens exercise, program leaders defended its importance by emphasizing that such research can drive future initiatives and priorities for caregivers, dispel misconceptions about caregivers across various organizations, and build a better understanding of the needs of specific groups. Three program leaders added that pursuing this research could clarify confusion about caregiver populations, noting, "the more we know, the better we can serve." The RGF panel added that caregivers of those who served in the military after 9/11 are young and, if not already married, will likely marry within the next five years, warranting a better understanding of the changing demographics and shifting needs of this population, as well as how to optimize services provided to this group.

Table 3.2
Median Panel Ratings, Site Plan Research Objectives

		Research Objective	
Dimension	Panel	Describe Caregivers	Quantify the Societal Cost Savings Attributed to Caregivers
Importance	Caregiver	Uncertain (6)	Important (8)
	RGF	Uncertain (6.5)	Important (8)
	Program leader	Important (7.5)	Important (7)
Effectiveness	Caregiver	Uncertain (5)	Uncertain (4.5)
	RGF	Effective (8)	Uncertain (6)
	Program leader	Uncertain (5)	Uncertain (5)
Cultural acceptability	Caregiver	Uncertain (5)	Uncertain (5)
	RGF	Acceptable (7)	Acceptable (7)
	Program leader	Uncertain (5)	Uncertain (5)
Implementation cost	Caregiver	Uncertain (4)	Uncertain (5)
	RGF	Uncertain (6)	Uncertain (6)
	Program leader	Uncertain (5)	Uncertain (5)
Learning potential	Caregiver	Uncertain (6)	High (8)
	RGF	Uncertain (6)	High (7)
	Program leader	Uncertain (6.5)	High (7)

Lastly, a caregiver noted that "communities want to accept the knowledge and understanding of [types of caregivers], but they have not been provided with accurate information," indicating that more research on this objective could prove to be worthwhile.

Overall, caregivers who participated in the ExpertLens panel emphasized that the caregiving population was too diverse to warrant research on the topic (one caregiver stated, "honestly, we are all so different") and that caregivers do not wish to be categorized based solely on their own characteristics or on the needs and demographics of their care recipients. Two caregivers additionally stated that research could do "the greatest good for the greatest number" by describing the characteristics of female, spousal caregivers. Another caregiver participant mentioned, in detail,

> Caregivers could be lumped into similar groups by [the] diagnosis they are caring for, but other characteristics that need to be looked at are the family aspects: how many children, their ages, education of the caregiver, employment of the caregiver. . . . The caregiver has had a lot of education on the topic, which could make the

caregiving easier, while another caregiver has not received the same amount of education. . . . I feel, as people, we want to be unique and not lumped into such categories as "this _____ kind of caregiver."

A potentially important theme of stigmatization as a caregiver emerged from rationales offered during the ExpertLens panel and from our observations and unstructured interviews of caregivers at the 2016 summit. Caregivers at the summit repeated that they have difficulty being forthright about their daily lives as caregivers and discussing taboo topics, such as sex and intimacy, financial issues, and their mental health or that of their care recipients. Participants in the program leader and caregiver panels added that many caregivers do not want to disclose their status as caregivers or reveal that their care recipient is affected by mental illness, which may further hinder progress on this research objective. Thus, stigma in this context is likely both self-imposed (e.g., shame) and interpersonal (e.g., being ostracized for a condition). While a more in-depth understanding of caregiver-related stigmatization is necessary, these findings may explain the lower cultural acceptability rating for this objective (median = 5/9 in the caregiver and program leader panels). This was echoed by a caregiver who noted, "I think there is still a silent stigma about caregiving, especially those of us with husbands between the ages of 20–40." In other words, the stigma, or shame, associated with caregiving may hinder the identification of different types of caregivers; however, this could also be interpreted as a motivating factor to perform research on this topic and help bring all who serve as caregivers out of the shadows.

Across all panels, those who rated the objective of describing caregivers to be of low importance and low learning potential commented that previous research had already addressed the various types of military and veteran caregivers. One RGF panel participant noted, "the issue is creating more awareness. There is already a ton of data with this information!" An important caveat to add is how often panel participants referenced previous RAND research, including the *Hidden Heroes* report, when evaluating this research objective. In total, five caregivers, two RGF panel participants, and four program leaders specifically mentioned RAND's work on describing and characterizing military and veteran caregivers. However, many cited it as a baseline for subsequent, more-detailed research. For example, one program leader stated, "The RAND study on the landscape of military and veteran caregivers was impressive and informative. A follow up and deeper dive may be a next step." In other words, existing research has likely provided a solid foundation that can be used to create more awareness and targeted interventions for all of the caregiving population.

Insights from the free-listing exercise and from observations and discussions at the summit help shed light on existing gaps in knowledge on the characteristics of military and veteran caregivers. In fact, the free-listing exercise elicited 11 specific types of caregivers whom individual participants considered to be important to study. Those types include caregivers who themselves serve in the military, children as caregivers, rural and isolated caregivers, caregivers for whom English is not a first language, male caregivers, caregivers with preexisting or chronic medical conditions, caregivers whose care recipient has died, aging parents as caregivers, caregivers who also have disabled children, college-aged caregivers, and caregivers of those who served in the military before 9/11. Although these types of caregivers may make up only a small portion of the broader population of caregivers, it is imperative to appreciate the diversity among caregivers and to understand how this variation influences their experiences, needs, and well-being.

Changing Needs

When evaluating the research objective of describing caregivers, survey data gathered during the summit in September 2016 were also informative. In the survey, we asked respondents to indicate the relative level of importance of research that would "shine light on different types of caregivers and how they are uniquely impacted by caregiving." Figure 3.1 shows how survey respondents rated the relative importance of each type of caregiver. In our survey, about half of the respondents rated parents serving as caregivers, young children serving as caregivers, and men serving as caregivers to be a high research priority. Conversely, one-third or less of survey respondents rated adult children, same-sex partners, siblings, and friends/neighbors to be a high research priority. From our earlier study, however, we know that these individuals may represent a substantial portion of the military and veteran caregiver population. It is possible that these individuals were underrepresented at the summit.

Although the research objective to describe caregivers was not considered as high a priority as other objectives, it may be that existing research on this topic has provided a solid foundation from which to continue describing the evolving caregiver population, making this objective more feasible to address than others. However, other research objectives described in this blueprint, such as understanding the effects of caregiving on the children of caregivers, may be considered more pressing to address. Yet, as the demographics of caregivers change and the landscape of caregiving continues to shift, describing caregivers will remain an important task. Taken together, research in the next decade could consider emphasizing the burgeoning population of younger adult caregivers, male caregivers, and children who serve as caregivers, as well as how the population of caregivers is changing in tandem with broader demographic changes in the United States (e.g., caregivers for whom English is a not a first language).

Quantify the Societal Cost Savings Attributed to Caregivers

Societal Savings

Another aspect of understanding how military and veteran caregivers contribute to U.S. society is documenting their contributions. Examples include studies that describe the specific tasks caregivers perform, assess caregivers' impact on care recipients' outcomes and quality of life, and calculate the value of caregivers' efforts for society. Toward this

Figure 3.1
Survey Results on the Priority of Research on Various Caregiver Attributes

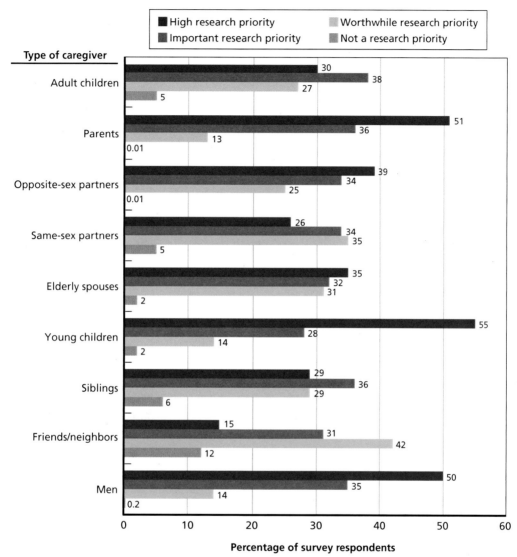

■ High research priority   ■ Worthwhile research priority
■ Important research priority   ■ Not a research priority

Type of caregiver

Adult children: 30, 38, 27, 5
Parents: 51, 36, 13, 0.01
Opposite-sex partners: 39, 34, 25, 0.01
Same-sex partners: 26, 34, 35, 5
Elderly spouses: 35, 32, 31, 2
Young children: 55, 28, 14, 2
Siblings: 29, 36, 29, 6
Friends/neighbors: 15, 31, 42, 12
Men: 50, 35, 14, 0.2

Percentage of survey respondents

end, our literature review revealed five publications relating to societal cost savings that can be attributed to efforts of caregivers. One article explored cost savings attributable to uncompensated, informal caregiving for dementia, one chapter was on Alzheimer's disease, and two articles explored cost savings attributed to elder caregiving in general. Estimates of cost saving fell between $159 billion and $215 billion annually for dementia to upward of $450 billion to $470 billion for elderly care. The sole publication that addressed cost savings attributed to military and veteran caregiving was the aforementioned 2014 RAND report, *Hidden Heroes: America's Military Caregivers*, which estimated the cost savings of the work of military and veteran caregivers at $14 billion annually (Ramchand, Tanielian, et al., 2014).

The identified published literature stresses the importance of understanding how characteristics of the caregiving population—especially demographic changes, including shrinking family sizes, an increasingly aging population, and increasing participation of women in the workforce—will change the landscape of cost savings attributed to caregiving. In addition, there is a need to understand the human costs of caregiving as they relate to societal cost savings, as well as cultural differences in the application of caregiving. Our literature review did not identify any articles that addressed societal cost savings attributed to military and veteran caregivers.

Although the $14 billion of cost savings estimated in RAND's 2014 report is high, the estimates represent an average of time lost across caregivers. Evaluating cost savings in the aggregate masks the unique attributes and needs of this population. In addition, time lost because of caregiving does not take into account additional burdens that caregivers face, such as a high prevalence of depression. Therefore, prior work has called for an understanding of cost savings in light of the costs of war and caregiving (e.g., health care costs, mental health burdens, lost workplace productivity) on society.

This research objective was rated as highly important across all three panels (median for caregiver and RGF panels = 8/9; for program leader panel = 7/9) with very high learning potential (median for caregiver panels = 8/9; RGF and program leader panels = 7/9). Panel participants consistently expressed their support, stating, "This is an extremely important research objective, as it will show society the real value of military and veteran caregivers in terms of dollars saved." They also added that such research would justify the costs of programs provided to caregivers and lend more support for additional research and programs for caregivers. That being said, the program leader panelists and caregivers rated the cultural acceptability of this objective to be uncertain (median = 5/9), while the RGF panelists rated it as acceptable (median = 7/9). Panelists elaborated on this by stating that fulfilling this research objective could raise awareness of caregivers and make tangible the benefits that caregivers bring to society. Lastly, one RGF panel participant made the case that collecting these data would be feasible, and the overall learning potential would be worth the investment.

Societal Costs

Across panels, participants noted that the research objective to quantify the societal cost savings attributed to caregivers should include not only such cost savings but also the costs that military and veteran caregivers must bear; that is, the objective should consider the *trade-offs* of caregiving. To this point, one caregiver noted,

> The better question is . . . what are the costs to society, as many veteran and nonveteran caregivers lose more money in ways of unearned income, which then impacts their Social Security benefits, and will then in turn [create] costs [to] soci-

ety. So, [are] there really cost savings attributed to caregiving? Perhaps in the short term for facilities, skilled nursing facilities, and such, but most definitely not to society as a whole.

Another caregiver noted,

> There is also the cost of losing your identity . . . When you meet people, almost the first question you get is, "What do you do for a living?" That is an emotional cost as well . . . and the general population does not realize just how important caregiving is.

Furthermore, one program leader admitted to being "torn" when rating the objectives because of the possibility that research will show that caregiving may not result in societal cost savings, which could detract from already depleted resources and programs available for caregivers and serve to limit support in the future.

Program leaders who rated this research objective as less important to pursue noted that extensive data are already being documented among other caregiver populations and that providing a definitive value of cost savings will not alter the status of military and veteran caregiving. Another program leader voiced the concern that this would be an important priority for policymakers but not to individual caregivers. The latter point suggests that while this research objective may help shape policy, caregivers may not see a direct and immediate benefit from the findings.

Despite these potential shortcomings, quantifying the cost savings attributed to informal, uncompensated caregiving of current and former service members is an important research objective to pursue, especially considering the scant literature on the topic and the simple fact that caregivers provide a societal benefit that too often goes unrecognized. In addition to weighing the costs and savings of informal caregiving, it is important to understand how they will be affected by the expanding population of care recipients and the demographic changes in U.S. society.

Overall, caregivers may not experience direct benefits of pursuing these research objectives in their daily lives; however, understanding who military and veteran caregivers are and the benefits they convey to society can help justify and guide programs and policies for caregivers that would lead to a more direct impact. In addition, broader societal changes, such as demographic shifts, are likely to affect who is able to serve as a caregiver. The fact that the existing evidence base does not adequately quantify the future cost savings attributed to military and veteran caregivers highlights the extent to which this is a gap. While the evidence base on describing caregivers broadly is more robust, literature on the range of military and veteran caregivers is scant and in need of more attention. Most importantly, fulfilling these research objectives can help build greater societal awareness and appreciation for caregivers of U.S. military veteran service members.

The Floor Plan

We define the floor plan of the caregiving research blueprint to include research that examines how caregiving impacts caregivers and their well-being. Of the ten research objectives, five fall within this category: Document the effects of caregiving on caregiver outcomes, assess the consequences of caregiving on the children of caregiving, document the effects of caregiving on care recipient outcomes, assess how the needs of care recipients change over time, and examine factors associated with caregiver and care recipient harm.

Document the Effects of Caregiving on Caregiver Outcomes

The literature review revealed 71 publications that investigated the impact of caregiving on caregivers: 53 focused on short-term outcomes (e.g., fatigue, anxiety, depression, divorce, disruption to work or school schedules, disruption to childcare, mental and physical health), and 18 focused on long-term outcomes (e.g., morbidity, health care utilization, income). Table 3.3 describes the evidence base of this research. Overall, there are more studies that have examined the impact of caregiving for individuals with dementia than there are for those caring for individuals with conditions more common among military and veteran caregivers, such as brain injury and mental illness. There are no studies on the long-term impact of caregiving specifically on military and veteran caregivers.

During our ExpertLens process to evaluate the research objectives, all three panels rated research on the consequences of caregiving on caregivers as very important (median for caregiver and program leader panels = 9/9; for RGF panel = 8/9) and with very high learning potential (median for caregiver panel = 9/9; for RGF and program leader panels = 8/9); see Table 3.4 for all panel ratings in the floor plan. However, only 49 percent of survey participants rated the consequences of caregiving as a high, important, or worthwhile research priority (51 percent rated it as not being a priority). The discrepancy may be partially explained by comments raised in the RGF panel, in which participants claimed that "this was well covered in *Hidden Heroes*" and "perhaps more is known here than for some other topics."

Nonetheless, two themes emerged across all the panels to highlight why continued research in this area is important. First, better understanding the impact of caregiving on caregivers could help inform programs and policies designed to mitigate any adverse effects. Second, caregivers reported that research could help them "tell their story." One caregiver noted, "It takes a multitude of problem-solving skills with very little time and total aggravation in trying to educate others what it's like" to be a caregiver. Another said, "I think more public education is needed on top of public awareness."

Table 3.3
Breakdown of Literature Examining the Short-Term and Long-Term Impacts of Caregiving on Caregivers

	Short-Term Impacts	Long-Term Impacts
Total	53	18
Type of publication		
Journal article	52	18
Book or report	1	0
Population		
Civilian	48	18
Military/veteran	5	0
Condition		
Dementia/Alzheimer's	19	4
Musculoskeletal injury	5	1
Heart disease	5	2
Stroke	3	0
Cancer	7	1
Brain injury	0	0
Paralysis	0	0
Burn	0	0
Mental illness	2	2
General elder care	4	2
Other	8	6

During the survey, we asked respondents "From your own perspective, please indicate the level of importance for the following outcomes associated with caregiving." Figure 3.2 shows the proportion of attendees who rated the various outcomes (quality of life, mental health, physical health, finances, families, intimate relationships) as a high, important, or worthwhile research priority or not a research priority. More attendees (77 percent) reported the mental health consequences of caregiving as highly important than any other outcome we asked about, although all the outcomes were highly endorsed. Next, we review these topics briefly in turn, including positive outcomes and potential barriers described by panelists.

Table 3.4
Median Panel Ratings, Floor Plan Research Objectives

Dimension	Panel	Document the Effects of Caregiving on Caregiver Outcomes	Assess the Consequences of Caregiving on the Children of Caregivers	Document the Effects of Caregiving on Care Recipient Outcomes	Assess How the Needs of Care Recipients Change over Time	Examine Factors Associated with Caregiver and Care Recipient Harm
Importance	Caregiver	Important (9)	Important (9)	Important (9)	Important (8)	Important (7)
	RGF	Important (8)	Important (9)	Important (9)	Important (8)	Important (7)
	Program leader	Important (9)	Important (9)	Important (8)	Important (8)	Important (7)
Effectiveness	Caregiver	Uncertain (4)	Uncertain (4)	Uncertain (5)	Uncertain (4.5)	Uncertain (4)
	RGF	Effective (7)	Uncertain (6)	Effective (7)	Uncertain (6)	Uncertain (3.5)
	Program leader	Uncertain (5)	Uncertain (4)	Uncertain (5)	Uncertain (5)	Uncertain (4)
Cultural acceptability	Caregiver	Uncertain (5)	Uncertain (6)	Uncertain (6.5)	Uncertain (5)	Uncertain (4)
	RGF	Acceptable (7)	Acceptable (8)	Uncertain (6)	Acceptable (8)	Uncertain (3.5)
	Program leader	Acceptable (7)	Acceptable (7)	Uncertain (5)	Uncertain (5)	Uncertain (5)
Implementation cost	Caregiver	Uncertain (4)	Uncertain (4.5)	Uncertain (4)	Uncertain (4)	Uncertain (4)
	RGF	Uncertain (4)	High (3)	Uncertain (4)	Uncertain (3)[a]	Uncertain (5)
	Program leader	Uncertain (5)	Uncertain (5)	Uncertain (4)	Uncertain (4)	Uncertain (5)
Learning potential	Caregiver	High (9)	High (9)	High (8)	High (7)	High (7)
	RGF	High (8)	High (8)	High (8)	High (7.5)	High (7)
	Program leader	High (8)	High (8)	High (7)	High (7)	High (7)

[a] This rating was categorized as uncertain due to disagreement within the panel. For all such ratings, see Table B.2 in Appendix B.

Figure 3.2
Survey Results on the Priority of Research on Various Caregiving Outcomes

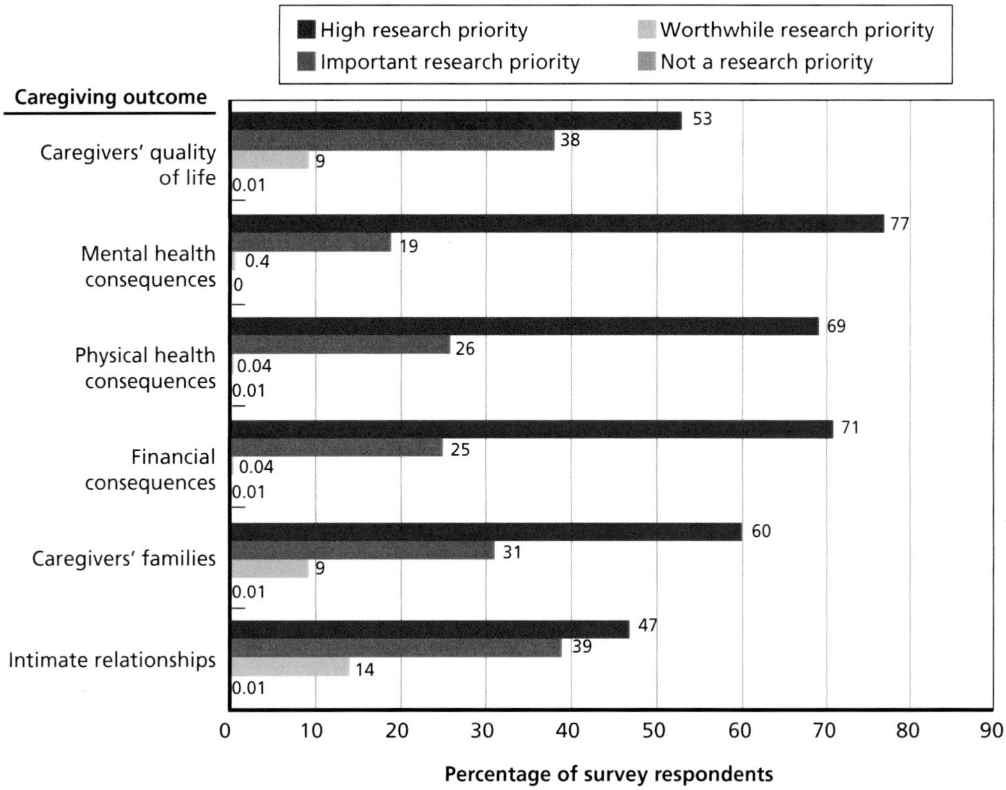

RAND RR1873-3.2

Mental and Physical Health Consequences

Caregivers in our panels spoke primarily about the stress-associated conditions and mental health outcomes related to caring for service members or veterans with mental health disorders. "I have seen trauma due to being someone's caregiver," said one, while another revealed, "I've also been diagnosed with an autoimmune disorder that is triggered by stress. I also have depression and anxiety." Another listed alcoholism, drugs, chronic health problems, depression, fibromyalgia, fatigue, and suicide as the "topics among caregivers in my circle."

Program representatives generally agreed that, for documenting the effects of caregiving on caregiver outcomes, "mental health figures in highly," while others spoke of health care utilization—for example, doctor's visits, time off from work, preventive care visits, and medication used. Others spoke of the importance of measuring such factors as weight and sleep, in addition to practicing healthy habits, such as eating a balanced diet and exercising.

Financial Consequences

The economic consequences discussed by panelists were primarily related to employment, but their comments reveal important nuances. Many spoke of "loss of work." Said one, "Hate that I had to give up a wonderful job for the most amazing company that worked with me, supported me in my employment as long as they could. But it felt horrible the day I packed up my desk and walked away." For some, loss of job meant loss of income and the pleasures associated with it, like travel or hiring someone to help with household chores. But for others, the income from working was a necessity: "The caregiver is torn between trying to make money to help make ends meet and also satisfying the demands of a potentially overwhelming role." Members of the RGF panel gave ideas about how these outcomes could be operationalized, suggesting "return to work" and "economic security" as outcomes to study.

Another aspect of employment that emerged from caregivers was missed or constrained employment opportunities because of caregiving duties. "Not pursuing more desired employment because [of] the caregiving role," "not furthering education to obtain a desirable job," and "not taking that desirable job because the hours are not doable while caregiving" were all mentioned by caregivers.

Effects on Caregivers' Families

Panelists raised several outcomes associated with family functioning. Among spouse caregivers, the outcomes ranged from marital strain to divorce and abuse. Said one caregiver about another caregiver she knew,

> It seems to me that the recipient ends up resenting the help that a spouse gives (much more so than a parent or sibling)—maybe because it emasculates them (as there is such a higher percentage of male wounded warriors than female), and they end up being abusive—verbally seems to be the most common form, but there are physical times too. No one should live with that, and some caregivers will leave if it comes to the spouse or their children being safe (they usually put themselves on the back burner, but their children take precedence over the wounded warrior most times); divorce seems to be high.

The other topic frequently raised, as exemplified by the panelist's comment, is how caregiving affects the relationship between a caregiver and his or her child. We discuss these outcomes as a separate research objective, but it is worth mentioning the struggle that some caregivers feel with respect to childcare, which is often tied to the loss of income addressed earlier. As one panelist stated,

> For spouses that have to give up jobs, they often have small children (and there seems to be a disproportionate number of special-needs kids with this generation of warriors) and will still need childcare to make the wounded warriors' doctor appointments—but with no way to pay for that (especially for those that don't live near family that will help out).

The impact of caregiving on families can also accumulate over time, and new stresses may emerge as caregivers and care recipients age. According to one caregiver,

> Although our children are grown (we've been married 34 years), it's exhausting when we have the grandchildren over because I have to not only watch them, but how my husband is responding to them. We are constantly on the edge of a fight unless we are sitting quietly. I'm exhausted always being on alert and I feel like my brain is going to implode. This is no way to continue living and this is not what we planned for in the autumn years of our marriage. We might not make it to our winter together.

Positive Outcomes

Although most panelists raised negative or adverse outcomes, the comment of one caregiver is worth including: "As I read the other participant comments, I would like to say that there can also be positive consequences while the question only mentions negative consequences." Thus, there is a need for studies to document the full range of impacts of caregiving, both positive and negative.

Potential Barriers

When discussing barriers to studying the effects of caregiving on caregivers, some caregivers reported that they may not be "completely honest and open about their needs" or that "they, themselves, may not have been aware of their needs." Another panelist echoed this sentiment:

> I think recognizing the depth of the needs is difficult because it forces us to accept the raw reality of our Hero's injuries. It brings a feeling of vulnerability and fear inside me, because acquaintances often flee when we share the reality of our lives. This abandonment makes me hesitant to accept any type of shoulder to lean on. The struggle is real. It's about a constant quest for balance and yet such an overwhelming feeling of being misunderstood and alone.

Assess the Consequences of Caregiving on the Children of Caregivers

As opposed to a somewhat voluminous literature examining how caregiving affects caregivers, our literature review revealed no research documenting the impact of caregiving on caregivers' children (see Table 3.5). Perhaps because of this, all three stakeholder groups (caregivers, RGF, and program leaders) rated research on the impact on children to be very important (the median rating for all three groups = 9/9), and all three also rated the learning potential to be high (median for caregiver panels = 9/9; for RGF and program leader panels = 8/9). Many caregivers wrote about their personal anecdotes stressing the importance of this type of research; said one, "I know that my children have had negative consequences as a result of my caregiving, so this assessment really has some validity."

Table 3.5
Breakdown of Literature Examining the Consequences of Caregiving on the Children of Caregivers, How Care Recipient Needs Change over Time, and Factors Associated with Caregiver or Care Recipient Harm

	Number of Sources Assessing the Consequences of Caregiving on the Children of Caregivers	Number of Sources Assessing How the Needs of Care Recipients Change over Time	Number of Sources Examining Factors Associated with Caregiver and Care Recipient Harm
Total	0	2	3
Type of publication			
Journal article	0	1	2
Book or report	0	1	1
Population			
Civilian	0	1	3
Military/veteran	0	1	0
Condition			
Dementia/Alzheimer's	0	1	0
Musculoskeletal injury	0	1	0
Heart disease	0	0	1
Stroke	0	0	0
Cancer	0	0	0
Brain injury	0	1	0
Paralysis	0	0	0
Burn	0	0	0
Mental illness	0	0	0
General elder care	0	0	1
Other	0	0	1

The perspectives shared by panelists on this topic yielded several, interrelated research areas: children serving as caregivers, the impact of being a child in a home with someone (usually a parent) who serves as a caregiver to someone with a mental health issue, and the impact of caregiving on parenting and the associated effect on children. Panelists also expressed concerns about the time horizon for these types of research studies, noting a need for studies of both short-term and long-term effects on children. In addition, many spoke about the cultural acceptability of conducting such research.

Children Serving as Caregivers

Of the summit survey respondents, 83 percent indicated that research on young children serving as caregivers was either a highly important or important research priority. A member of the program panel, when discussing services available to caregivers, suggested that there is a notable gap in services for children serving as caregivers. One caregiver told us, "Our children seem to be the forgotten secondary caregivers."

Children of Caregivers to Persons with a Mental Health Condition

Members of the caregiver panel (as opposed to the other panels) primarily raised the topic of children living in homes in which caregivers (usually their parents) are caring for someone with a mental health condition. This topic often overlapped with issues related to parenting, discussed next. For example, one caregiver told us, "It is hard explaining [the] behavior of a spouse that isn't good behavior due to a [traumatic brain injury]." Another revealed something similar:

> These kids . . . (this question made my eyes fill with tears). The kids are growing up every day caught in the middle of a life that is so hard to understand as an adult, much less for a child. They do not understand why they cannot participate in extracurricular activities. Mommy doesn't know if Daddy will have a bad day and need her at a moment's notice, and there will be missed games, practices, etc. Or what if Daddy has an outburst in front of the other families?

Another caregiver echoed this sentiment:

> School for dependents of wounded warriors can be hard because they can't have a "normal" childhood—too many can't have friends come stay, they have to tiptoe around a parent that has numerous triggers for posttraumatic stress, there is possible emotional and/or physical abuse in their home.

Effects of Caregivers' Parenting on Children

Caregivers frequently brought up the issue of the competing roles of caring for the care recipient and caring for their children. A caregiver spouse told us,

> Because the caregiver job is so demanding, the children have less than half of the mother that I once aspired to be. It breaks my heart to the depths of my soul. All I ever wanted was to be married to this man and raise his babies. I'm thankful for the dreams that have come true, but in the midst of coping with the brokenness, I see even more falling apart around me. I listen to audio tapes in hopes to self-improve, to find better ways to make myself stretch all the way around. I know in my head it isn't possible and that I'm doing the best that I can, but my heart—my heart hurts for the children. They are growing up so fast while I am busy trying to be whatever my veteran needs me to be.

Some provided more-specific examples about the aspects of parenting that are affected by caregiving. For example, some care recipients compete for attention. One caregiver indicated, "My child is grown, but I know when she is around, I can barely get a normal conversation with her because of all the attention my veteran needs." Another caregiver spoke about not meeting societal expectations that may exist for parents: "People still don't seem to understand why I have the limitations to do certain things like go on a field trip in my kid's classroom." And finally, a caregiver who is caring for her 27-year-old son receives criticism from her other son who "feels that I am coddling his brother and there is resentment. Truth to tell, I have no idea if this is normal sibling issues or how much has to do with what I have to do to help my oldest."

Short-Term Effects

Program leaders were most vocal about describing some of the short-term outcomes worth examining for research on the impact of caregiving on children. The following five broad categories were mentioned:

- school performance (e.g., grades, missed days of school/sick days, class participation)
- attachment issues (e.g., codependency)
- socialization (e.g., participation in extracurricular activities, isolation, friends, play group, being bullied, participation within the family)
- adverse behaviors (e.g., bullying, substance seeking, reckless behavior, aggression, drugs and alcohol use)
- mental health (e.g., depression, anxiety, stress).

Long-Term Effects

Across all groups, many panelists discussed the need for research on the long-term impacts of caregiving on children. "I'd love to see a study done on the impact [on] adult children," one caregiver wrote, revealing that her children "were in middle school when this all began and now they have children of their own. And yes, I do think that has had an effect on their parenting and relationship status." In general, the panelists were not very specific about what outcomes they would want to see researched, but one caregiver said that "health, mental well-being, and identity are at risk."

Related to long-term outcomes, one panelist suggested examining postsecondary school choices—"Do they stay or do they go?" Across these outcomes, a panelist from the program leader group provided examples specific to ages for which an outcome is most appropriate, separating young children, preteens, and teens. Although mental health outcomes may not exhibit themselves until later in a child's development, two panelists suggested the need to examine "emerging behavioral or mental health issues" that may be reflected in young children's behaviors.

It was in discussing the long-term effects that many participants, particularly from the program leader and RGF panels, highlighted the need for longitudinal research, which they knew would be costly. Members of the program leader panel commented, "Need longitudinal research—it will be expensive," and "A longitudinal study may cost a lot, but would be important." Members of the RGF panel provided more detail with respect to costs; one stated, "this line of research is no more expensive than other social science studies exploring stressors and resource needs of special populations. The issue is access to subjects/participants, which may increase recruitment costs." Thus, while the caregiver and program leader panelists were uncertain about the costs of assessing how caregiving affects children (where 1 was expensive and 9 was not expensive, caregiver median = 4.5/9; program leader median = 5/9), the RGF group rated this research objective as expensive to implement (median = 3/9).

Cultural Acceptability Issues

The panels differed somewhat on the cultural acceptability of conducting research on the impact of caregiving on children (median score for caregiver panel = 6/9; RGF = 8/9; program leader = 7/9). In their comments, caregivers provided insights not mentioned by program leader and RGF panelists. For example, caregivers noted that some parents would be unwilling to share insights about their children because they may feel it would be criticized. Said one caregiver, "some families may NOT want their children divulging family 'secrets'—for example, how much they may help, or that a parent may be scary at times." Another agreed: "I think some caregivers would be very sensitive about this topic—potentially feeling like their parenting skills are being judged."

Document the Effects of Caregiving on Care Recipient Outcomes

In addition to the focus on how caregiving affects caregivers and their children, the effects of caregiving on care recipient outcomes was identified as an area of research interest. The literature review revealed 36 articles addressing this topic, primarily examining short-term outcomes (28) rather than long-term outcomes (8) (see Table 3.6). All three panels rated research on this topic as important and as having high learning potential.

Several panelists commented that documenting the effects of caregiving on care recipient outcomes was important as a means to justify programs and support services for caregivers. One caregiver noted, "Concrete evidence on the benefits of caregiving could help fiscally justify supporting caregivers." Another said, "If there was more research and documentation on the impact of caregiving on veterans, I believe there would also be greater community support and funding for services and programs to help veterans and caregivers." This theme was echoed by a member of the RGF panel, who noted, "We need to be able to show [the benefit of caregiving for care recipient outcomes] to make the case for continued and increased funding." Furthermore, program leaders commented, "This would be useful in designing programs for support," and "If resources are to be increased that are targeted to caregivers, there must be strong evidence of need and impact." One program leader summed it up as follows: "We are in

Table 3.6
Breakdown of Literature Examining the Short-Term and Long-Term Impacts of Caregiving on Care Recipient Outcomes

	Short-Term Impacts	Long-Term Impacts
Total	28	8
Type of publication		
Journal article	28	8
Book or report	0	0
Population		
Civilian	26	8
Military/veteran	2	0
Condition		
Dementia/Alzheimer's	3	1
Musculoskeletal injury	0	0
Heart disease	7	0
Stroke	0	0
Cancer	7	1
Brain injury	0	1
Paralysis	0	0
Burn	0	0
Mental illness	2	0
General elder care	0	2
Other	9	3

an outcomes-driven world. Documenting the outcomes is critical." Thus, panel members saw this research question as important to justify continued support for programs and services for caregivers.

This research topic was rated as having high learning potential, and comments from caregivers reinforced the potential for gains in knowledge (e.g., "Potential for learning is limited only by the scope of the study"). A few caregivers reiterated that research on how caregivers can be trained to better help care recipients has learning potential: "We can learn the best caregiving practices and more-effective training can be developed." When asked the types of outcomes that the research should focus on, one RGF panelist mentioned return to work, volunteer, quality of life, economic security, and happiness; another panelist agreed with the list and added community engagement and family functioning. The program leader panel added physical health—doctor's visits, time off from work, preventive care visits, weight, sleep, and medication used.

Several RGF panel members commented that a lot is already known about this question, so the learning potential may be less than that for other questions. One RGF panelist commented, "This might take some longer-term study, but reviewing what we already know and using surveys to fill in gaps can give us a good amount of info immediately." Another suggested that new directions for this research would add to the knowledge gained: "We need to learn better ways to improve the mental health and quality of life of military families." Similarly, a program leader panelist commented specifically on the potential knowledge gained from studying caregivers of post-9/11 service members: "We need to start building the baseline of knowledge. After 15 years of war, we have post-9-11 vets and their caregivers at multiple stages in their journey—we can learn a lot." Although it is true that more research has been published on this topic than on the other topics related to this research objective, panel members noted that there are still gaps in knowledge that could be addressed by future research.

Ratings of effectiveness, cultural acceptability, and implementation cost were mixed. Caregiver and program leader panels were uncertain about the effectiveness of prior research, but RGF participants rated prior research as effective (median rating = 7/9). One RGF panelist noted, "More is known here" and commented that "I'm not sure how 'special' the [military/veteran] space is in terms of needing distinct knowledge." Regarding research on military and veteran caregivers, another RGF panelist wrote, "Related studies date back to earlier wars, which have shown that learning about the impact of caregiving on veterans is vital to reducing costs at all levels." Another RGF panelist acknowledged the previous research in this area and noted, "Too many cross-sectional studies have been conducted in the past. It is time to fund longitudinal studies using a randomized controlled design so we can be doing meta-analysis on effectiveness studies."

All three panels were uncertain about the cultural acceptability of research on the impact of caregiving on care recipient outcomes (median ratings from 5/9 to 6/9). Panelist comments suggested that this uncertainty was partly because the cultural acceptability was "unknown." Other comments suggested that this topic may be culturally acceptable but that acceptability was counterbalanced by concerns about the stigma associated with caregiving. An RGF panelist noted that this topic was "possibly sensitive—caregivers may not want to reveal problems," and another noted the "'stigma' associated with the caregiving role." Several caregivers echoed the perception of stigma around caregiving. For example, one caregiver commented, "I think it's still culturally taboo to talk about caregiving, especially those of us with younger husbands." Another caregiver noted, "some caregivers may feel like they are being judged for how well their care impacts their recipient." One program leader sounded a hopeful note by commenting, "I think it is becoming more culturally relevant and especially as the population of caregivers diversifies and is given faces."

Panelists were also uncertain about the implementation costs of this research question (for all panels, median rating = 4/9). Comments generally reflected the theme that "this depends on the type of study to be done. More rigor and adequate population size require more resources" (program leader). RGF panelists noted, "It is very expensive to do well-designed efficacy studies," and the studies "might require physical exams, longitudinal follow up, etc." Other, less-expensive options were suggested by caregivers: "Studies are being done; should be easy to piggyback off of them." However, one caregiver commented, "You get what you pay for. A good study needs an appropriate amount of resources to complete, which includes time and money."

Assess How the Needs of Care Recipients Change Over Time

Our review of the literature found only two studies that examined how care recipient needs change over time, and all three panels rated this research question as important (median ratings for all three panels = 8/9), with high learning potential (median ratings for the caregiver and program leader panel = 7/9; RGF panel = 7.5/9). Several panelists commented that it is especially important to begin doing this research with post-9/11 care recipients now. For example, one RGF panelist noted, "Our post-9/11 veterans are generally young, and their needs will likely become more complex and demanding as they age." Others commented that it is important that research is conducted so that caregiver skills and knowledge keep pace with the changes in care recipient needs over time: "Too often, change in [activities of daily living] performance is not addressed and, consequently, dyads are performing [such activities] unsafely or without proper [training]." A couple of program leaders noted that studies might need to distinguish the long-term needs of different populations; one stated, "I suspect this will be very individualized—changes probably vary greatly by type of injury, type of care, and myriad factors."

The effectiveness of prior research on this topic was rated as uncertain by all panels (median ratings ranged from 4.5/9 to 6/9). One RGF panelist noted, "There is a big database of research on older veterans that addresses at least some of these issues," possibly referring to studies of the health care needs of Vietnam and Gulf War veterans. However, several panelists lamented the "lack of longitudinal studies on the care needs of veterans and caregivers," noting that this "area is still very understudied and consequently poorly supported."

RGF panelists rated this question as culturally acceptable (median rating = 8/9), but program leaders and caregivers rated cultural acceptability as uncertain (both panels' median rating = 5/9). One program leader commented, "I am not sure whether it is cultural acceptability or taking the caregivers for granted or as having an obligation to give care." A few caregivers noted that the cultural acceptability of this question might vary depending on whether the population studied was pre-9/11 or post-9/11 service members. One caregiver commented that there needed to be a focus on Vietnam veterans and not just post-9/11 veterans because "Vietnam vets are also needing more care as they age because of war-related injuries or exposures." Another caregiver questioned whether "people (general population) are more accepting that a Vietnam-era veteran needs long-term care than [that] a post-9/11, or even Desert Storm, veteran" does. One caregiver responded,

> I think that society is more accepting of a Vietnam-era veteran needing care than a post-9/11 [veteran]. I always assumed that it had to do with the recipient's age. The idea of a Hero in their 20s and 30s needing a caregiver seems overwhelming and expensive long-term because they are so "young." Also, there is the idea that "the young bounce back faster."

Finally, all three panels rated the implementation cost of this question as uncertain but trended to the cost being more expensive (median ratings ranged from 3/9 to 4/9). Several participants from all three panels agreed that research in this area "would have to be focused on longitudinal studies," which are "so much more resource intense."

Examine Factors Associated with Caregiver and Care Recipient Harm

Three articles examined harm and fraud related to caregiving. This could include interpersonal abuse (caregiver on care recipient or vice versa), as well as abuse of benefits and programs by caregivers or care recipients (referred to as fraud). Median ratings of importance and learning potential for this research objective were high for all three stakeholder types (all panels' median ratings = 7/9 for both dimensions). One RGF panelist noted, "We know from research with civilian populations that care recipient harm is more rampant that we estimate, so this area definitely deserves attention." A program leader said, "There are anecdotal stories of harm, but we need to lift the curtain on what actually is happening," and another commented, "Many caregivers are subjected to hidden abuse by their Veterans—mostly emotional." Several program leaders noted the benefit of learning more about this research objective, commenting that the results could be put to use to "create warning signs for advocates to identify" and could "shape actions in the medical community (to avoid caregiver harm)." One program leader summed up the potential of this objective by noting, "I believe we can actually make a huge difference in five years by adding this research goal into the mix."

Given the few studies we found in our literature search, it is not surprising that all three panels rated the prior effectiveness of research on this topic as uncertain (median ratings ranged from 3.5/9 to 4/9). RGF and program leader panelists expressed that they "think the literature is quite limited in this area," and "In the past, I think [research] has been anecdotal, not integrated among sources of information."

Despite the general agreement that this is an important topic with high learning potential, there was a lively discussion among members of all three panels about the cultural acceptability of this research objective (median ratings ranged from 3.5/9 to 5/9). RGF and program leader panelists commented on the difficulty of measuring harm and fraud when it is "very difficult to get honest answers about abuse." Still, several program leaders offered ideas for how to conduct this research in a culturally acceptable manner. One program leader commented that "caregivers would self-report if they felt something positive would come from it," but the panelist also felt that "funding sources other than VA, who already have [intimate partner violence] coordinators, will be challenging since this is an 'unpleasant' topic and some feel stats [of abuse or fraud] are inflated. They are not." Another noted that

> the method of gathering data and conveying to caregivers that their information is confidential/protected—building a platform for data collection that is viewed as a safe place—may likely help. As a caregiver of both a young and older generation, answering some of these questions in a safe environment would be a relief for some who may feel very isolated.

Caregivers generally echoed these comments. One noted,

> This is a very difficult area to research and get honest answers, because caregivers abusing or perpetrating fraud are not going to self report, and the most fragile care recipients may not be able or willing to report (or they may be unaware of fraud). And many caregivers who are being abused by the veteran are ashamed to admit it has gotten to that point, or they believe they can handle the situation, or they have been providing care and have few "safe" options [for] themselves or their veteran.

There was some disagreement among program leaders and caregivers about whether there is a potential disincentive for having the care recipient's health improve, because it could result in losing caregiver benefits. Panelists commented, "I don't think the majority of caregivers would want anything but improvement of their care recipient," and "There will be some in the category who take advantage of benefits, but by and large, and from my experience, that is the exception rather than the rule." But several expressed a different view. For example, one stated, "Disability is enabled by providing a stipend for that disability. It's very difficult to take something away, particularly income, when the veteran does get better." Caregivers commented that "our care recipient may have good days and bad days, but downplaying improvements I don't see happening." Other caregivers noted the potential conflict. For example, one stated,

> Yes, there is a potential disincentive for having the care recipient's health improve. Care recipient improvement is a catch-22, meaning that if the care recipient improves, the caregiver loses financial support and most likely must secure full-time employment. Going back to full-time employment for the caregiver increases stress in the household and also increases the likelihood that the care recipient's health will decline. My care recipient would most likely not take his medicine,

participate in his own health care, exercise, eat nutritiously, or inquire about his health really at all without my constant supervision. I'm not sure what the solution is here, but this is where I am at this moment. Losing benefits is very frightening to me not only because of my husband's health, but mine as well.

Finally, panelists rated the implementation cost of research on caregiver or care recipient harm as uncertain (median ratings ranged from 4/9 to 5/9). RGF panelists noted, "I'm not sure expense and difficulty correspond, but the difficulty level is definitely high," and "Given fear and privacy concerns, this area of research will likely require creative studies that may cost more than expected." Program leader panelists suggested that "studies could link in with other consumer protection investigations," or the research could incorporate "record investigation and interviewing" to cut costs. One program leader commented that the research would be "too expensive to justify large costs."

The Elevation

For the elevation piece in our research blueprint, we explore those research objectives that examine how external forces impact caregivers. Namely, we focus on studies that assess how various interventions, whether at the program or policy level, affect caregiver and other outcomes.

An important component of research designed to improve support for military and veteran caregivers relates to examining the *efficacy* (i.e., whether an intervention has the intended impact under ideal circumstances, such as in an experiment) and *effectiveness* (i.e., whether an intervention has the intended impact in more-usual or real-world conditions) of existing caregiving interventions. The literature review revealed 84 publications focused on this topic. These covered the following five areas:

- improvements to the accessibility of caregiver programs
- effectiveness of programs in ensuring caregiver well-being (e.g., evaluations of respite services, workplace flexibility)
- effectiveness of health care policies supporting caregivers (e.g., revisions to privacy laws, changes to screening procedures)
- effectiveness of programs and policies supporting caregivers' ability to provide care (e.g., education, training, knowledge, technology)
- effectiveness of workplace policies supporting caregivers (e.g., flexible work schedules).

For the most part, caregiver interventions examined effectiveness in real-world settings, although several interventions examined efficacy in a clinical or randomized trial setting (e.g., Cheng et al., 2014; Limiñana-Gras et al., 2016). For simplicity, we use the term *effectiveness* in our discussion here, but these results are pertinent to caregiver interventions in all types of settings—clinical, randomized control trials, and real world.

The vast majority of research was on the effectiveness of programs and policies supporting caregivers' ability to provide care; such programs included those providing informal and formal education and training, assessments of caregiver knowledge and information programs, and programs using new technologies (e.g., telehealth, smartphones) to assist caregivers with caregiving tasks. Our review turned up only a handful of studies on interventions to improve the accessibility of caregiver programs and no studies on the effectiveness of workplace policies to support caregivers, despite caregivers often reporting the need for such interventions. The lack of studies on workplace intervention could be a consequence of the search criteria we used, but the fact that we found no studies at all suggests that this is an area ripe for future interventions.

About one-third of the literature on the effectiveness of programs and policies for ensuring caregiver well-being and supporting caregivers' ability to provide care focused on the population of care recipients with dementia. Interventions related to the accessibility of caregiver programs have much more diversity in terms of the disease condition of the care recipient. Table 3.7 describes the existing research on caregiver interventions based on our review of the literature.

Identify Strategies for Making Effective Programs Accessible to More Caregivers

In the general discussions about identifying strategies for making effective programs accessible to more caregivers, the RGF panel suggested that social media would be the most effective way to reach caregivers. Yet, caregivers suggested a broader variety of ways to find out about programs—for example, through social media, word of mouth, sporting events, retreats, peer support networks, and Internet searches. Panelists voiced concern about listservs or emails as a method of relaying information, stating that there is generally too much information provided, much of which is not pertinent. Caregivers called for a better way to provide relevant, targeted information to caregivers about existing interventions.

Table 3.8 shows the median panel ratings emerging from our ExpertLens process concerning the effectiveness of interventions. Identifying strategies for making effective programs accessible to more caregivers was rated as highly important by all panels (median for all panels = 9/9), with high learning potential (median for all panels = 8/9). As one caregiver succinctly put it, "If caregivers can't access the programs, what is the point of having the program? [This] makes it very important."

With respect to the other dimensions (effectiveness, cultural acceptability, and implementation cost), ratings varied greatly (median rating hovered around 5/9 or 6/9). Panelists generally had little to no knowledge about implementation costs, with some voicing concern that a program might be costly but justified, given the potential impact. For the most part, the panels had similar median ratings, with the exception

Table 3.7
Breakdown of Literature Examining the Efficacy and Effectiveness of Caregiver Interventions

	Accessibility of Caregiver Programs	Effectiveness of Programs Ensuring Caregiver Well-Being	Effectiveness of Programs and Policies Supporting Caregivers' Ability to Provide Care		
			Health Care Policies	Workplace Policies	Other Programs
Total	10	24	12	0	38
Type of publication					
Journal article	10	23	11	0	35
Book or report	0	1	1	0	3
Population					
Civilian	9	21	8	0	32
Military/veteran	1	3	4	0	6
Condition					
Dementia/Alzheimer's	0	8	2	0	13
Musculoskeletal injury	1	1	0	0	0
Heart disease	2	1	2	0	1
Stroke	0	1	0	0	1
Cancer	0	2	2	0	6
Brain injury	0	0	0	0	2
Paralysis	0	0	0	0	0
Burn	0	0	0	0	0
Mental illness	1	2	0	0	4
General elder care	1	2	0	0	2
Other	5	7	6	0	9

of cultural acceptability, which was rated as acceptable (median rating = 7/9) from the RGF panel but as uncertain (6/9) from the caregiver and program leader groups. It is worth noting that although the median rating among caregivers was uncertain overall, there was a lot of variability in the scores. Some caregivers on the panel did not perceive any concerns about cultural acceptability. Others felt that there was a lack of cultural acceptability. The reasons for this were summed up by one caregiver: "I think that, ideologically, people support caring for veterans. Practically speaking, many are cynical when that care is rendered by spouses or family members . . . [and] view it in practice as sort of a government handout."

Table 3.8
Median Panel Ratings, Elevation Research Objectives

Dimension	Panel	Identify Strategies for Making Effective Programs Accessible to More Caregivers	Evaluate the Effectiveness of Programs and Policies for Ensuring Caregiver Well-Being	Identify Effective Programs and Policies to Support Caregivers' Ability to Provide Care
Importance	Caregiver	Important (9)	Important (9)	Important (9)
	RGF	Important (9)	Important (8)	Important (9)
	Program leader	Important (9)	Important (9)	Important (8)
Effectiveness	Caregiver	Uncertain (5)	Uncertain (5)	Uncertain (4)
	RGF	Uncertain (5.5)	Uncertain (5)	Effective (7)
	Program leader	Uncertain (4.5)	Uncertain (4)	Uncertain (5)
Cultural acceptability	Caregiver	Uncertain (6)	Uncertain (5)	Uncertain (6)
	RGF	Acceptable (7)	Acceptable (7)	Uncertain (6)
	Program leader	Uncertain (6)	Uncertain (5)	Uncertain (5)
Implementation cost	Caregiver	Uncertain (5)	Uncertain (5)	Uncertain (5)
	RGF	Uncertain (5)	High (3.5)	Uncertain (5)
	Program leader	Uncertain (5)	Uncertain (5)	High (3)
Learning potential	Caregiver	High (8)	High (8)	High (8)
	RGF	High (8)	High (7)	High (8)
	Program leader	High (8)	High (8)	High (8)

Evaluate the Effectiveness of Programs and Policies for Ensuring Caregiver Well-Being

Caregivers voiced several concerns that existing programs to ensure caregiver well-being, while accessible, may not always be available. Said one caregiver, "Is access the same as availability? I think a caregiver could have access to a program but not have the program available to them because there may be a waiting list, or when the caregiver needs the program, it is not open." In addition, concerns were raised that caregivers may eschew such interventions because they suggest that the caregivers cannot handle their responsibilities. As one caregiver noted, "Utilizing such services could be looked at as though the caregiver can't handle their situation and are pawning it off on someone else." These comments suggest other potential limitations to program access that need to be addressed to ensure that caregiver well-being programs are truly available and acceptable.

Despite these concerns, all three panels rated the effectiveness of programs and policies for ensuring caregiver well-being as highly important, with high learning potential. One of the main reasons cited multiple times for the importance of this topic related to "caregiver burden" or "burnout." This is a theme that is noted in the research literature and was voiced by participants on all three panels. Program leader and RGF participants further pointed out the link between caregiver and care recipient well-being, as indicated by a program leader: "If we don't take care of ourselves, there will be no energy to take care of our veterans."

Although there was agreement that this topic is important, once again, effectiveness, cultural acceptability, and cost had median ratings of "uncertain," for the most part. The one exception was the RGF panel, which rated this objective as culturally acceptable (median = 7/9). RGF panelists also provided lower ratings for implementation costs (median = 3.5/9) than did the other groups (median = 5/9). Comments suggested that implementation costs were expected to be high, but as one RGF participant stated, although there is investment on the front end, it "pays for itself."

Identify Effective Programs and Policies to Support Caregivers' Ability to Provide Care

Identifying effective programs and policies supporting caregivers' ability to provide care was similarly rated by all panels as highly important, with high learning potential. This topic elicited many comments about how caregivers are often thrown into care with little knowledge of where to turn for guidance. One caregiver summarized, "I really do not see any of this in place at all. A lot of times it feels like we are on our own." Another noted, "Most people are not born a caregiver. We require information [for what our] loved one or the person we are caring for is going through."

Panelists cited caregiver burnout as a reason for the significance of interventions for caregiver well-being. However, other panel discussions raised another type of fatigue—bureaucracy fatigue—which relates more directly to caregiver training needs on how to navigate organizations. Some members of the program leader panel discussed this further. Said one, "caregivers already have so much on their 'plate,' and then [have] to face a disorganized organization that requires numerous calls, not understanding benefits, and rotating providers." Another followed up on this point, claiming that "'bureaucracy fatigue' [is] consequential and debilitating to even the most stalwart caregiver."

As with the other types of caregiving interventions evaluated by the panels, effectiveness of the intervention, cultural acceptability, and implementation cost were rated as uncertain by all panels. One exception was the effectiveness dimension, which was rated effective (median = 7/9) by the RGF panel but rated lower by the caregiver and program leader panels. While some of the caregivers cited the *Hidden Heroes* report as showing that past studies pursuing this research objective have been effective, many caregivers voiced concerns that most programs are not well known and, thus, their effectiveness may be unknown. As one caregiver noted, "I don't think they've been terribly effective because there remain little resources and too many veterans, caregivers, and their families [who] are suffering due to limited and lacking resources."

Most of the program panelists said that they were unaware of studies on the effectiveness of programs or policies to support caregivers' ability to provide care. One member of the program leader panel summed this up as follows:

> I think we've been more in "identifying the needs" mode rather than what's work-ing. It's time to move beyond simple need identification in order to bring clarity to program developers and caregivers on what is most effective. This is even more important now because so many different organizations (government and non-profit) are entering the "caregiver support" space. How is a caregiver supposed to know what resource is best for them?

The panelists' ratings of the potential implementation costs varied widely by group and dimension. For example, the program leader panel rated this objective as high cost (median = 3/9); the median score for the other panels was rated uncertain (median = 5/9).

The findings from the ExpertLens process were complemented by survey responses. During the survey, we asked respondents to indicate the relative importance of vari-ous types of efforts for caregivers (e.g., evaluating existing programs for caregivers, implementing research-based programs for caregivers in real-world settings). Respon-dents rated each category as a high, important, or worthwhile research priority or not a research priority. Implementing research-based programs for caregivers in real-world settings (58 percent) and evaluating the benefits of existing programs on caregiver well-being (55 percent) were rated as high priorities by the largest percentage of attendees. Slightly fewer than half of the attendees rated the other areas for intervention as high priorities. This is consistent with the panel discussions, in which all the topics posed were rated as important. Figure 3.3 shows these results.

To summarize, within the elevation piece of our research blueprint, we used a combination of information gleaned about effectiveness and, to a lesser extent, efficacy of interventions from the stakeholder panels, ExpertLens data, survey, and literature review. The expert panels unanimously rated all three of the research objectives in this piece as important. This was confirmed by the survey data as well.

On the effectiveness, cultural acceptability, and implementation cost dimensions, agreement was less clear. Most of the panelists rated effectiveness and implementation costs as unknown. Ratings of cultural acceptability were uncertain at the median as well, but this was a result of the vast range of scores rather than because individual attendees were uncertain. The individual scores for this dimension often ranged from 2/9 to 9/9, with attendees in the same panels having vastly different opinions about the acceptability of these research objectives.

The literature review also revealed several gaps in the relevant academic and policy literature. There were few studies on interventions related to accessibility of care and none related to workplace policies. While our search terms may not have included all studies in this area, the paucity of evidence suggests that the effectiveness and effects

Figure 3.3
Survey Results on the Priority of Research on Various Caregiver Interventions

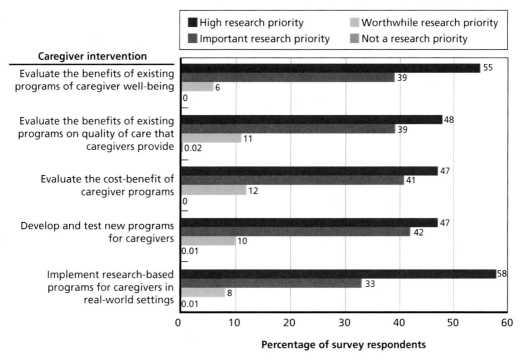

RAND RR1873-3.3

of workplace interventions for caregivers may be an area ripe for future work. The ExpertLens panels suggested that little is known about the effectiveness of programs for caregiver training, and members of all panels stated that they were aware of only limited work in this area.

It is worth noting that the RGF panel ratings were sometimes inconsistent with those of the other two panels. This may suggest that the available research has not permeated the consciousness of the general public or program stakeholders. Further efforts may be needed to translate academic findings on the effectiveness of interventions so that they may be accessible to other stakeholders, including, importantly, family caregivers.

Cross-Cutting Issues

Across the research objectives we reviewed and assessed, there were several issues that can be viewed as cutting across all three of our blueprint plans. Many of these issues result from the lack of studies on specific subpopulations of caregivers. Stakeholders identified two subpopulations of specific interest: men and children. Studies focused on these populations should go beyond just describing who the caregivers are (a research objective listed in the site plan) and extend to research objectives that examine how caregiving affects them in ways that may be unique or different from the impact experienced by women or spouses (populations that make up the majority of the literature discussed in the floor plan). Also needed are studies that assess the efficacy and effectiveness of programs or policies for these specific groups (as outlined in the elevation).

Stakeholders also expressed concern about the lack of studies focused on those caring for a particular type of care recipient, particularly those who experienced a brain injury or related mental health disorder. Our literature review confirmed the dearth of studies focused on caregivers for individuals with these conditions. We note, however, that there is currently a large longitudinal study being implemented by the Department of Defense to study the caregivers of service members who experienced a traumatic brain injury during the post-9/11 era. This study, which has yet to publish any findings, represents a significant investment, but additional research will still be needed on this subpopulation over time to ensure that the full range of issues affecting caregivers is examined.

Limitations and Caveats

While we sought to use research methods that are efficient for gathering multiple types of data and that offer the least burden and time constraints, there are limitations intrinsic to the study design. First, the literature review was limited in two ways. The time frame of publications may have missed information collected on caregivers of pre-9/11 service members prior to 2005, which could have been beneficial in illustrating key differences among present-day caregivers. In addition, the inventory of existing research excluded that based outside the United States. This may have omitted insights from caregiving research among military and veteran families in other contexts, such as studies conducted in the United Kingdom. Furthermore, our literature review did not include a quality assessment or a risk of bias assessment of the included publications.

Second, the convenience sample used for the initial survey findings, while diverse, may not be representative of all stakeholders and experts on military and veteran caregiving. It is highly likely that caregivers and other advocates who attended the Elizabeth Dole Foundation summit differ from the wider population of military and veteran caregivers. For example, some of the subgroups of military and veteran caregivers (e.g., those supporting individuals pre-9/11) may have been underrepresented. This may, in turn, raise concerns about the generalizability of our findings.

Furthermore, as is the case with other versatile, web-based Delphi platforms, ExpertLens has limitations. One is that it assumes participants will form their ratings based on the responses and feedback of other participants, but it is difficult to know whether they, in fact, do. Our sample of caregivers who participated in an ExpertLens panel may also not be representative of the broader population of military and veteran caregivers. This could be attributed to the fact that participants would need to have Internet access, be Internet savvy, have seen the announcement posted by the Elizabeth Dole Foundation on Twitter (excluding those who are not Twitter users), and have time to contribute to the study. There may have also been questions of interpretation or a lack of clarity on the proposed research objectives and the dimensions on which they were evaluated. Also, an inherent risk of bias is that participants may have simply conformed to the median ratings without critically evaluating their opinions and the judgment of other participants. And because ExpertLens provides median ratings, it may not adequately address the range of ratings. In addition, because we did not collect respondent characteristics before each round, there is no means of adequately testing for any statistically significant differences among respondents and nonrespondents. Lastly, the attrition rate across panels was high, indicating that final ratings may not adequately reflect those of the overall panel.

This study reflects a particular snapshot within the ever-changing context of caregiving. That is to say, the political climate, the demands placed on the military, the challenges to the health and well-being of care recipients, the funding and programs available to caregivers, and the visibility and prioritization of caregiving and military families in society are in a constant state of flux. Hence, the research priorities described in this report may become more or less pressing in future years, making this point less of a limitation and more of a call to keep issues of caregiver well-being at the forefront of U.S. priorities.

Summary of Stakeholder Ratings

Table 3.9 aggregates what we learned from all panels of our stakeholder consensus process about the importance of a specific research objective, the effectiveness of previous research on that topic, the cultural acceptability of conducting research in that area, the implementation cost of performing new research, and the learning potential of new research in this area over the next five years. For this summary table, we converted all of the ratings into the same scale of high (instead of important, effective, or acceptable), uncertain, or low to enable comparison across the dimensions. This table also highlights the number of published articles identified for each of the objectives, enabling a view of potential gaps and areas for future investment.

Table 3.9
Summary of Median Ratings Across Stakeholder Panels

Focus (Blueprint Component)	Research Objective	Importance	Effectiveness	Cultural Acceptability	Implementation Cost	Learning Potential	Number of Articles Identified[a]
Caregivers as members of society (site plan)	Describe caregivers.	Uncertain*	Uncertain*	Uncertain*	Uncertain	Uncertain	34 (5)
	Quantify the societal cost savings attributed to caregiving.	High	Uncertain	Uncertain*	Uncertain	High	5 (1)
Impacts of caregiving on caregivers, care recipients, and their families (floor plan)	Document the effects of caregiving on caregiver outcomes.	High	Uncertain*	Uncertain	Uncertain	High	72 (6)[b]
	Assess the consequences of caregiving on the children of caregivers.	High	Uncertain	High	Uncertain*	High	0 (0)
	Document the effects of caregiving on care recipient outcomes.	High	Uncertain*	High**	Uncertain	High	36 (0)
	Assess how the needs of care recipients change over time.	High	Uncertain	Uncertain*	Uncertain	High	2 (1)
	Examine factors associated with caregiver and care recipient harm.	High	Uncertain	Uncertain	Uncertain	High	3 (0)

Table 3.9—Continued

Focus (Blueprint Component)	Research Objective	Importance	Effectiveness	Cultural Acceptability	Implementation Cost	Learning Potential	Number of Articles Identified[a]
External factors that influence caregiving (elevation)	Identify strategies for making effective programs available to more caregivers.	High	Uncertain	Uncertain*	Uncertain	High	10 (1)
	Evaluate the effectiveness of programs and policies for ensuring caregiver well-being.	High	Uncertain	Uncertain*	Uncertain*	High	24 (3)
	Identify effective programs and policies to support caregivers' ability to provide care.	High	Uncertain*	Uncertain	Uncertain	High	50 (10)

NOTE: The color shading is used to distinguish the median ratings. High is shaded in blue, and uncertain is in gray. For the number of articles, red reflects areas where there is a gap in research, and green reflects areas with an abundance of published research.

* One panel rated this as high.

** One panel rated this as uncertain.

[a] The number in parentheses represents the number of articles that specifically focused on military or veteran caregivers.

[b] Griffin et al. (2016) is included in this table but was published after our literature review was complete; therefore, that research is not necessarily reflected in our analysis of the literature in other sections of the report.

CHAPTER FOUR

Strategies to Consider for Using the Blueprint

As we noted in Chapter One, the role of this blueprint is to convey a vision for future research that will build support for military and veteran caregivers. In essence, the blueprint becomes a guide for the community to use in prioritizing and facilitating future research. It is not a manual for how research should be pursued; stakeholders may use the blueprint differently as they craft their own specific activities. Caregivers and their advocates can use the blueprint as a reference point to encourage funding organizations to expand research opportunities in each of the areas outlined. The funding community can use the blueprint as a reference or guide to creating research priorities for allocating their research budgets. As researchers design future studies, they can refer to the blueprint as a source of stakeholder-endorsed research objectives. Ideally, the blueprint becomes a mechanism and common reference point for the various stakeholder communities to work toward a common goal of improving support for military and veteran caregivers by conducting rigorous research.

To ensure that the blueprint can become a central feature of and motivator for future research, we outline three potential strategies for how to gain support, adoption, and implementation of the blueprint.

Establish Partnerships

To be maximally effective in implementing the blueprint, the military and veteran caregiver stakeholder community can partner with other organizations with interests in research on caregivers or caregiving issues. There are a wide array of organizations and entities that have a vested interest in expanding the research base on caregiving, and this blueprint joins other recent reports calling for increased research to improve programs and policies that support caregivers.

For example, the National Academies of Science, Engineering, and Medicine's Committee on Family Caregiving for Older Adults released a report in September 2016 outlining recommendations aimed at addressing the health, economic, and social issues facing family caregivers of older Americans (National Academies of Sciences, Engineering, and Medicine, 2016). Many of these recommendations are relevant for military and veteran caregivers as well, partly because many of the nation's veterans are part of the "older adult" population; furthermore, many of the recommendations are appropriate regardless of the age of the care recipient. Among the committee's recommendations, several call for the testing and evaluation of new programs, policies, or other mechanisms that serve to identify caregivers, assess their needs, and ensure that they are engaged appropriately in health care delivery processes. The recommendations also call for testing or evaluating interventions designed to support caregivers and assessing policies that provide economic support for working caregivers. Most notably, the committee called for the VA and the U.S. Department of Health and Human Services to create a public-private, multistakeholder innovation fund for research and innovation to accelerate the pace of change in addressing the needs of caregiving families. The research objectives that we evaluated and arrayed in this blueprint can all be nested within these larger objectives and used as a basis for informing how the VA and Department of Defense in particular can support and implement this recommendation.

The National Academies report provides an opportunity to position this blueprint within a larger stakeholder community and perspective. Another recent report outlined a research agenda on a specific type of caregiver support program—respite care—and can be used to provide much more detail for the elevation piece outlined in this report. In 2015, the ARCH (Access to Respite Care and Health) National Respite Network and Resource Center released *A Research Agenda for Respite Care: Deliberations of an Expert Panel of Researchers, Advocates and Funders* (Kirk and Kagan, 2015). The respite care research agenda in that report can serve as somewhat of a template for how to conceptualize evaluations of other caregiver support or caregiver intervention programs. Kirk and Kagan specifically outlined the need to research a wide variety of outcomes (individual, family, and societal) associated with respite care and to conduct appropriate cost-benefit and cost-effectiveness research (which would fall within our floor and elevation plans, respectively). The respite care research agenda also called for studies examining system changes that improve access to such care (an issue that we identified as a component of the elevation) and that would help inform policy and practice through translational research.

Beyond efforts to integrate this blueprint with other existing research agendas, the stakeholder community could forge additional partnerships and consortia with other caregiver organizations to call for increased research funding, catalyze the research community to focus on caregiving, and demand more evidence-based decisionmaking for future caregiver support programs and policies. Following the completion of its research plan, the ARCH National Respite Network and Resource Center put forth a prospectus for a Respite Research Funding Consortium, which could serve as both a model for the military and veteran caregiver community and a source of support for funding some of the research objectives in this blueprint.

Convene a Military and Veteran Caregiver Research Summit

Another opportunity to promote awareness and facilitate progress toward implementation would be to host a research summit focused specifically on cultivating new research studies designed around the blueprint components. Such a summit could bring together researchers from across disciplines, potential funders, and caregiver representatives to help refine research questions and discuss research design ideas and funding opportunities. Ideally, the summit conveners could gain some commitment from potential funding organizations that would be willing to commit resources to new studies. The summit could be modeled after such summits as the VA's State of the Science in Traumatic Brain Injury in 2015 but could place a high priority on working sessions designed to outline specific studies for each of the research objectives in this blueprint.

Create a Research Center of Excellence

Facilitating innovation and advances in research in military and veteran caregiving can also be accomplished by creating a dedicated research center of excellence. Centers of excellence can be used to help build capacity, foster innovation and best practices across a field, develop new knowledge, and speed translation and dissemination into practice and policy. The U.S. government has used research centers of excellence in several fields of study to ensure appropriate infrastructure, management, and capacity to jumpstart and maintain a stream of research in a given area. Within the military and veteran caregiving community, the designation of a research center of excellence or research collaborative could help foster the strategic pursuit of the research blueprint and fill the existing knowledge gaps outlined in this report, thus helping to ensure better support for military and veteran caregivers in the future.

Bibliography

Adelman, Marcy, "Overcoming Barriers to Care for LGBT Elders with Alzheimer's," *Generations,* Vol. 40, No. 2, Summer 2016.

Agren, S., A. Stromberg, T. Jaarsma, and M. L. Luttik, "Caregiving Tasks and Caregiver Burden; Effects of an Psycho-Educational Intervention in Partners of Patients with Post-Operative Heart Failure," *Heart Lung*, Vol. 44, No. 4, July–August 2015, pp. 270–275.

Andruszkiewicz, Grace, and Katy Fike, "Emerging Technology Trends and Products: How Tech Innovations Are Easing the Burden of Family Caregiving," *Generations*, Vol. 39, No. 4, Winter 2015/2016.

Apesoa-Varano, Ester Carolina, Yajarayma Tang-Feldman, Susan C. Reinhard, Rita Choula, and Heather M. Young, "Multi-Cultural Caregiving and Caregiver Interventions: A Look Back and a Call for Future Action," *Generations*, Vol. 39, No. 4, Winter 2015/2016.

Avieli, Hila, Sarah Ben-David, and Inna Levy, "Predicting Professional Quality of Life Among Professional and Volunteer Caregivers," *Psychological Trauma: Theory, Research, Practice, and Policy*, Vol. 8, No. 1, 2016, pp. 80–87.

Avsar, U., U. Z. Avsar, Z. Cansever, A. Yucel, E. Cankaya, H. Certez, M. Keles, B. Aydinli, and N. Yucelf, "Caregiver Burden, Anxiety, Depression, and Sleep Quality Differences in Caregivers of Hemodialysis Patients Compared with Renal Transplant Patients," *Transplantation Proceedings*, Vol. 47, No. 5, June 2015, pp. 1388–1391.

Bailey, Whitney A., and Sarah R. Gordon, "Family Caregiving Amidst Age-Associated Cognitive Changes: Implications for Practice and Future Generations," *Family Relations*, Vol. 65, No. 1, February 2016, pp. 225–238.

Bakas, T., J. K. Austin, B. Habermann, N. M. Jessup, S. M. McLennon, P. H. Mitchell, G. Morrison, Z. Yang, T. E. Stump, and M. T. Weaver, "Telephone Assessment and Skill-Building Kit for Stroke Caregivers: A Randomized Controlled Clinical Trial," *Stroke*, Vol. 46, No. 12, December 2015, pp. 3478–3487.

Bassal, Catherine, Judith Czellar, Susanne Kaiser, and Elise S. Dan-Glauser, "Relationship Between Emotions, Emotion Regulation, and Well-Being of Professional Caregivers of People with Dementia," *Research on Aging*, Vol. 38, No. 4, May 2016, pp. 477–503.

Beharie, N., M. C. Lennon, and M. McKay, "Assessing the Relationship Between the Perceived Shelter Environment and Mental Health Among Homeless Caregivers," *Behavioral Medicine*, Vol. 41, No. 3, 2015, pp. 107–114.

Bejjani, Carla, A. Lynn Snow, Katherine S. Judge, David M. Bass, Robert O. Morgan, Nancy Wilson, Annette Walder, Wendy J. Looman, Catherine McCarthy, and Mark E. Kunik, "Characteristics of Depressed Caregivers of Veterans with Dementia," *American Journal of Alzheimer's Disease and Other Dementias*, Vol. 30, No. 7, 2015, pp. 672–678.

Bekhet, Abir K., "Resourcefulness in African American and Caucasian American Caregivers of Persons with Dementia: Associations with Perceived Burden, Depression, Anxiety, Positive Cognitions, and Psychological Well-Being," *Perspectives in Psychiatric Care*, Vol. 51, No. 4, 2015, pp. 285–294.

Bernard, Brittany L., Lauren E. Bracey, Kathleen A. Lane, Denisha Y. Ferguson, Michael A. LaMantia, Sujuan Gao, Douglas K. Miller, and Christopher M. Callahan, "Correlation Between Caregiver Reports of Physical Function and Performance-Based Measures in a Cohort of Older Adults with Alzheimer Disease," *Alzheimer Disease and Associated Disorders*, Vol. 30, No. 2, 2016, pp. 169–174.

Biggar, A., and A. Hood, "The Complex Landscape of Family Caregiving," *Generations*, Vol. 39, No. 4, 2015.

Black, Kathy, "Establishing Empirically-Informed Practice with Caregivers: Findings from the CARES Program," *Journal of Gerontological Social Work*, Vol. 57, No. 6–7, 2014, pp. 585–601.

Blair, Judith, Marie Volpe, and Brooke Aggarwal, "Challenges, Needs, and Experiences of Recently Hospitalized Cardiac Patients and Their Informal Caregivers," *Journal of Cardiovascular Nursing*, Vol. 29, No. 1, 2014, pp. 29–37.

Block, Cady, Katherine Fabrizio, Beau Bagley, Joanna Hannah, Susan Camp, Nazaren Mindingall, Don Labbe, and Kristine Lokken, "Assessment of Veteran and Caregiver Knowledge About Mild Traumatic Brain Injury in a VA Medical Center," *Journal of Head Trauma Rehabilitation*, Vol. 29, No. 1, 2014, pp. 76–88.

Blumenthal-Barby, J. S., K. M. Kostick, E. D. Delgado, R. J. Volk, H. M. Kaplan, L. A. Wilhelms, S. A. McCurdy, J. D. Estep, M. Loebe, and C. R. Bruce, "Assessment of Patients' and Caregivers' Informational and Decisional Needs for Left Ventricular Assist Device Placement: Implications for Informed Consent and Shared Decision-Making," *Journal of Heart and Lung Transplantation*, Vol. 34, No. 9, September 2015, pp. 1182–1189.

Brank, Eve M., and Lindsey E. Wylie, "Differing Perspectives on Older Adult Caregiving," *Journal of Applied Gerontology*, Vol. 35, No. 7, July 2016, p. 698.

Buchanan, Robert J., Chunfeng Huang, and Adele Crudden, "Use of the Internet by Informal Caregivers Assisting People with Multiple Sclerosis," *Journal of Technology in Human Services*, Vol. 30, No. 2, 2012, pp. 72–93.

Buck, H. G., J. Mogle, B. Riegel, S. McMillan, and M. Bakitas, "Exploring the Relationship of Patient and Informal Caregiver Characteristics with Heart Failure Self-Care Using the Actor-Partner Interdependence Model: Implications for Outpatient Palliative Care," *Journal of Palliative Medicine*, Vol. 18, No. 12, December 2015, pp. 1026–1032.

Buhse, Marijean, Carol Della Ratta, Janet Galiczewski, and Patricia Eckardt, "Caregivers of Older Persons with Multiple Sclerosis: Determinants of Health-Related Quality of Life," *Journal of Neuroscience Nursing*, Vol. 47, No. 2, 2015, pp. E2–E12.

Bull, Margaret J., Lesley Boaz, and Jennifer M. Sjostedt, "Family Caregivers' Knowledge of Delirium and Preferred Modalities for Receipt of Information," *Journal of Applied Gerontology*, Vol. 35, No. 7, July 2016, pp. 744–758.

Bunn, Frances, Claire Goodman, Emma Pinkney, and Vari M. Drennan, "Specialist Nursing and Community Support for the Carers of People with Dementia Living at Home: An Evidence Synthesis," *Health and Social Care in the Community*, Vol. 24, No. 1, January 2016, pp. 48–67.

Burton, Allison M., Jessica M. Sautter, James A. Tulsky, Jennifer Hoff Lindquist, Judith C. Hays, Maren K. Olsen, Sheryl I. Zimmerman, and Karen E. Steinhauser, "Burden and Well-Being Among a Diverse Sample of Cancer, Congestive Heart Failure, and Chronic Obstructive Pulmonary Disease Caregivers," *Journal of Pain and Symptom Management*, Vol. 44, No. 3, 2012, pp. 410–420.

Camak, D. J., "Addressing the Burden of Stroke Caregivers: A Literature Review," *Journal of Clinical Nursing*, Vol. 24, No. 17–18, September 2015, pp. 2376–2382.

Casado, Banghwa Lee, Sang E. Lee, Michin Hong, and Seokho Hong, "The Experience of Family Caregivers of Older Korean Americans with Dementia Symptoms," *Clinical Gerontologist,* Vol. 38, No. 1, January 2015, pp. 32–48.

Casida, J., H. S. Wu, J. Harden, A. Carie, and J. Chern, "Evaluation of the Psychometric Properties of Self-Efficacy and Adherence Scales for Caregivers of Patients with a Left Ventricular Assist Device," *Progress in Transplantation*, Vol. 25, No. 2, June 2015, pp. 116–123.

Chan, K. Y., T. Yip, D. Y. Yap, M. K. Sham, Y. C. Wong, V. W. Lau, C. W. Li, B. H. Cheng, W. K. Lo, and T. M. Chan, "Enhanced Psychosocial Support for Caregiver Burden for Patients with Chronic Kidney Failure Choosing Not to Be Treated by Dialysis or Transplantation: A Pilot Randomized Controlled Trial," *American Journal of Kidney Disease*, Vol. 67, No. 4, April 2016, pp. 585–592.

Cheak-Zamora, Nancy C., and Michelle Teti, "'You Think It's Hard Now… It Gets Much Harder for Our Children': Youth with Autism and Their Caregiver's Perspectives of Health Care Transition Services," *Autism: The International Journal of Research and Practice*, Vol. 19, No. 8, November 2015, pp. 992–1001.

Chen, L. F., J. Liu, J. Zhang, and X. Q. Lu, "Non-Pharmacological Interventions for Caregivers of Patients with Schizophrenia: A Meta-Analysis," *Psychiatry Research*, Vol. 235, January 30, 2016, pp. 123–127.

Chen, Mei-Lan, "The Growing Costs and Burden of Family Caregiving of Older Adults: A Review of Paid Sick Leave and Family Leave Policies," *Gerontologist*, Vol. 56, No. 3, June 2016, pp. 391–396.

Cheng, Sheung-Tak, "Double Compression: A Vision for Compressing Morbidity and Caregiving in Dementia," *Gerontologist*, Vol. 54, No. 6, December 2014, pp. 901–908.

Cheng, Sheung-Tak, Rosanna W. L. Lau, Emily P. M. Mak, Natalie S. S. Ng, and Linda C. W. Lam, "Benefit-Finding Intervention for Alzheimer Caregivers: Conceptual Framework, Implementation Issues, and Preliminary Efficacy," *Gerontologist*, Vol. 54, No. 6, December 2014, pp. 1049–1058.

Christensen, Janelle J., and Heide Castaneda, "Danger and Dementia: Caregiver Experiences and Shifting Social Roles During a Highly Active Hurricane Season," *Journal of Gerontological Social Work*, Vol. 57, No. 8, 2014, pp. 825–844.

Claassen, C. A., J. L. Pearson, D. Khodyakov, P. M. Satow, R. Gebbia, A. L. Berman, D. J. Reidenberg, S. Feldman, S. Molock, M. C. Carras, R. M. Lento, J. Sherrill, B. Pringle, S. Dalal, and T. R. Insel, "Reducing the Burden of Suicide in the U.S.: The Aspirational Research Goals of the National Action Alliance for Suicide Prevention Research Prioritization Task Force," *American Journal of Preventive Medicine*, Vol. 47, No. 3, 2014, pp. 309–314.

Clarke, Philip B., Jonathan K. Adams, Joseph R. Wilkerson, and Edward G. Shaw, "Wellness-Based Counseling for Caregivers of Persons with Dementia," *Journal of Mental Health Counseling*, Vol. 38, No. 3, 2016, pp. 263–277.

Coleman, E. A., K. L. Ground, and A. Maul, "The Family Caregiver Activation in Transitions (FCAT) Tool: A New Measure of Family Caregiver Self-Efficacy," *Joint Commission Journal on Quality and Patient Safety*, Vol. 41, No. 11, November 2015, pp. 502–507.

Corallo, F., L. Bonanno, S. De Salvo, A. Giorgio, C. Rifici, V. Lo Buono, P. Bramanti, and S. Marino, "Effects of Counseling on Psychological Measures in Caregivers of Patients with Disorders of Consciousness," *American Journal of Health Behavior*, Vol. 39, No. 6, November 2015, pp. 772–778.

Dalal, A. K., P. C. Dykes, S. Collins, L. S. Lehmann, K. Ohashi, R. Rozenblum, D. Stade, K. McNally, C. R. Morrison, S. Ravindran, E. Mlaver, J. Hanna, F. Chang, R. Kandala, G. Getty, and D. W. Bates, "A Web-Based, Patient-Centered Toolkit to Engage Patients and Caregivers in the Acute Care Setting: A Preliminary Evaluation," *Journal of American Medical Informatics Association*, Vol. 23, No. 1, January 2016, pp. 80–87.

Damme, Mary Jane, and Susan Ray-Degges, "A Qualitative Study on Home Modification of Rural Caregivers for People with Dementia," *Journal of Housing for the Elderly*, Vol. 30, No. 1, January/March 2016, pp. 89–106.

Danzl, Megan M., Anne Harrison, Elizabeth G. Hunter, Janice Kuperstein, Violet Sylvia, Katherine Maddy, and Sarah Campbell, "'A Lot of Things Passed Me by': Rural Stroke Survivors' and Caregivers' Experience of Receiving Education from Health Care Providers," *Journal of Rural Health*, Vol. 32, No. 1, Winter 2016, pp. 13–24.

Dunkle, Ruth E., Sheila Feld, Amanda J. Lehning, Hyunjee Kim, Huei-Wern Shen, and Min Hee Kim, "Does Becoming an ADL Spousal Caregiver Increase the Caregiver's Depressive Symptoms?" *Research on Aging*, Vol. 36, No. 6, November 2014, pp. 655–682.

Edwards, Megan, "Family Caregivers for People with Dementia and the Role of Occupational Therapy," *Physical and Occupational Therapy in Geriatrics*, Vol. 33, No. 3, 2015, pp. 220–232.

Eifert, Elise K., Rebecca Adams, William Dudley, and Michael Perko, "Family Caregiver Identity: A Literature Review," *American Journal of Health Education*, Vol. 46, No. 6, 2015, pp. 357–367.

Ejem, Deborah B., Patricia Drentea, and Olivio J. Clay, "The Effects of Caregiver Emotional Stress on the Depressive Symptomatology of the Care Recipient," *Aging and Mental Health*, Vol. 19, No. 1, 2015, pp. 55–62.

Engebretson, A., L. Matrisian, and C. Thompson, "Pancreatic Cancer: Patient and Caregiver Perceptions on Diagnosis, Psychological Impact, and Importance of Support," *Pancreatology*, Vol. 15, No. 6, November–December, 2015, pp. 701–707.

Ewing, J., "Supporting Family Caregivers," *NCSL Legisbrief*, Vol. 23, No. 10, March 2015, pp. 1–2.

Fauth, Elizabeth Braungart, Elia E. Femia, and Steven H. Zarit, "Resistiveness to Care During Assistance with Activities of Daily Living in Non-Institutionalized Persons with Dementia: Associations with Informal Caregivers' Stress and Well-Being," *Aging and Mental Health*, Vol. 20, No. 9, 2016, pp. 888–898.

Feinberg, Lynn Friss, and Carol Levine, "Family Caregiving: Looking to the Future," *Generations*, Vol. 39, No. 4, Winter 2015/2016, pp. 11–20.

Fitch, Kathryn, Steven J. Bernstein, Maria Dolores Aguilar, Bernard Burnand, Juan Ramon LaCalle, Pablo Lazaro, Mirjam van het Loo, Joseph McDonnell, Janneke Vader, and James P. Kahan, *The RAND/UCLA Appropriateness Method User's Manual*, Santa Monica, Calif.: RAND Corporation, MR-1269-DG-XII/RE, 2001. As of March 14, 2017:
http://www.rand.org/pubs/monograph_reports/MR1269.html

Fitts, W., D. Weintraub, L. Massimo, L. Chahine, A. Chen-Plotkin, J. E. Duda, H. I. Hurtig, J. Rick, J. Q. Trojanowski, and N. Dahodwala, "Caregiver Report of Apathy Predicts Dementia in Parkinson's Disease," *Parkinsonism and Related Disorders*, Vol. 21, No. 8, August 2015, pp. 992–995.

Ford, B. K., B. Ingersoll-Dayton, and K. Burgio, "Care Transition Experiences of Older Veterans and Their Caregivers," *Health and Social Work*, Vol. 41, No. 2, May 2016, pp. 129–138.

Francis, L. E., G. Kypriotakis, E. E. O'Toole, K. F. Bowman, and J. H. Rose, "Grief and Risk of Depression in Context: The Emotional Outcomes of Bereaved Cancer Caregivers," Omega (Westport), Vol. 70, No. 4, 2015, pp. 351–379.

Friedman, Esther M., Regina A. Shih, Kenneth M. Langa, and Michael D. Hurd, "US Prevalence and Predictors of Informal Caregiving for Dementia," *Health Affairs*, Vol. 34, No. 10, October 2015, pp. 1637–1641.

Fronczek, A. E., "A Phenomenologic Study of Family Caregivers of Patients with Head and Neck Cancers," *Oncology Nursing Forum*, Vol. 42, No. 6, November 2015, pp. 593–600.

Gage, Barbara, and Asmaa Albaroudi, "The Triple Aim and the Movement Toward Quality Measurement of Family Caregiving," *Generations*, Vol. 39, No. 4, Winter 2015/2016, pp. 28–33.

Ganapathy, V., G. D. Graham, M. D. DiBonaventura, P. J. Gillard, A. Goren, and R. D. Zorowitz, "Caregiver Burden, Productivity Loss, and Indirect Costs Associated with Caring for Patients with Poststroke Spasticity," *Clinical Interventions in Aging*, Vol. 10, 2015, pp. 1793–1802.

Gaugler, J. E., M. Reese, and M. S. Mittelman, "Effects of the Minnesota Adaptation of the NYU Caregiver Intervention on Depressive Symptoms and Quality of Life for Adult Child Caregivers of Persons with Dementia," *American Journal of Geriatric Psychiatry*, Vol. 23, No. 11, November 2015, pp. 1179–1192.

———, "Effects of the Minnesota Adaptation of the NYU Caregiver Intervention on Primary Subjective Stress of Adult Child Caregivers of Persons with Dementia," *Gerontologist*, Vol. 56, No. 3, June 2016, pp. 461–474.

Gaugler, Joseph E., Bonnie L. Westra, and Robert L. Kane, "Professional Discipline and Support Recommendations for Family Caregivers of Persons with Dementia," *International Psychogeriatrics*, Vol. 28, No. 6, 2016, pp. 1029–1040.

Gauthier, M. A., S. Cossette, M. F. Ouimette, and V. Harris, "Intervention for Advanced Heart Failure Patients and Their Caregivers to Support Shared Decision-Making About Implantation of a Ventricular Assist Device," *Canadian Journal of Cardiovascular Nursing*, Vol. 26, No. 2, Spring 2016, pp. 4–9.

Gelman, Caroline Rosenthal, Tracey Sokoloff, Noel Graziani, Emma Arias, and Anyelina Peralta, "Individually-Tailored Support for Ethnically-Diverse Caregivers: Enhancing Our Understanding of What Is Needed and What Works," *Journal of Gerontological Social Work*, Vol. 57, No. 6–7, 2014, pp. 662–680.

George, Nika R., and Ann Steffen, "Physical and Mental Health Correlates of Self-Efficacy in Dementia Family Caregivers," *Journal of Women and Aging*, Vol. 26, No. 4, 2014, pp. 319–331.

Gilmore-Bykovskyi, A. L., T. J. Roberts, B. J. Bowers, and R. L. Brown, "Caregiver Person-Centeredness and Behavioral Symptoms in Nursing Home Residents with Dementia: A Timed-Event Sequential Analysis," *Gerontologist*, Vol. 55, Supp. 1, June 2015, pp. S61–S66.

Gitlin, L. N., and K. Rose, "Impact of Caregiver Readiness on Outcomes of a Nonpharmacological Intervention to Address Behavioral Symptoms in Persons with Dementia," *International Journal of Geriatric Psychiatry*, Vol. 31, No. 9, September 2016, pp. 1056–1063.

Goldsmith, J., E. Wittenberg, C. S. Platt, N. T. Iannarino, and J. Reno, "Family Caregiver Communication in Oncology: Advancing a Typology," *Psychooncology,* Vol. 25, No. 4, April 2016, pp. 463–470.

Grebeldinger, T. A., and K. M. Buckley, "You Are Not Alone: Parish Nurses Bridge Challenges for Family Caregivers," *Journal of Christian Nursing,* Vol. 33, No. 1, January–March 2016, pp. 50–56.

Griffin, Joan M., Greta Friedemann-Sánchez, Kathleen F. Carlson, Agnes C. Jensen, Amy Gravely, Brent C. Taylor, Sean M. Phelan, Kathryn Wilder-Schaaf, Sherry Dyche Ceperich, and Courtney Harold Van Houtven, "Resources and Coping Strategies Among Caregivers of Operation Iraqi Freedom (OIF) and Operation Enduring Freedom (OEF) Veterans with Polytrauma and Traumatic Brain Injury," in Shelley MacDermid Wadsworth and David S. Riggs, eds., *Military Deployment and Its Consequences for Families,* New York: Springer Science + Business Media, 2014, pp. 259–280.

Griffin, J. M., M. K. Lee, L. R. Bangerter, C. H. Van Houtven, G. Friedemann-Sánchez, S. M. Phelan, K. F. Carlson, and L. A. Meis, "Burden and Mental Health Among Caregivers of Veterans with Traumatic Brain Injury/Polytrauma," *American Journal of Orthopsychiatry,* Vol. 87, No. 2, 2017, pp. 139–148.

Griffiths, Patricia C., M. Kate Whitney, and Mariya Kovaleva, "Development and Implementation of Tele-Savvy for Dementia Caregivers: A Department of Veterans Affairs Clinical Demonstration Project," *Gerontologist,* Vol. 56, No. 1, 2016, pp. 145–154.

Grossman, Brian R., and Catherine E. Webb, "Family Support in Late Life: A Review of the Literature on Aging, Disability, and Family Caregiving," *Journal of Family Social Work,* Vol. 19, No. 4, July/September 2016, pp. 348–395.

Han, Areum, and Jeff Radel, "Spousal Caregiver Perspectives on a Person-Centered Social Program for Partners with Dementia," *American Journal of Alzheimer's Disease and Other Dementias,* Vol. 31, No. 6, 2016, pp. 465–473.

Hendrix, C. C., D. E. Bailey, Jr., K. E. Steinhauser, M. K. Olsen, K. M. Stechuchak, S. G. Lowman, A. J. Schwartz, R. F. Riedel, F. J. Keefe, L. S. Porter, and J. A. Tulsky, "Effects of Enhanced Caregiver Training Program on Cancer Caregiver's Self-Efficacy, Preparedness, and Psychological Well-Being," *Support Care Cancer,* Vol. 24, No. 1, January 2016, pp. 327–336.

Henning-Smith, Carrie E., Gilbert Gonzales, and Tetyana P. Shippee, "Barriers to Timely Medical Care for Older Adults by Disability Status and Household Composition," *Journal of Disability Policy Studies,* Vol. 27, No. 2, September 2016, pp. 116–127.

Hernandez, Haniel, Joel Scholten, and Elsie Moore, "Home Clinical Video Telehealth Promotes Education and Communication with Caregivers of Veterans with TBI," *Telemedicine and e-Health,* Vol. 21, No. 9, 2015, pp. 762–766.

Hernandez, Mercedes, and Concepción Barrio, "Perceptions of Subjective Burden Among Latino Families Caring for a Loved One with Schizophrenia," *Community Mental Health Journal,* Vol. 51, No. 8, November 2015, pp. 939–948.

Hoagwood, Kimberly, and Serene S. Olin, "The NIMH Blueprint for Change Report: Research Priorities in Child and Adolescent Mental Health," *Journal of the American Academy of Child and Adolescent Psychiatry,* Vol. 41, No. 7, 2002, pp. 760–767.

Holden, Richard J., Christiane C. Schubert, and Robin S. Mickelson, "The Patient Work System: An Analysis of Self-Care Performance Barriers Among Elderly Heart Failure Patients and Their Informal Caregivers," *Applied Ergonomics,* Vol. 47, 2015, pp. 133–150.

Hong, Sung-Chull, and Constance L. Coogle, "Spousal Caregiving for Partners with Dementia: A Deductive Literature Review Testing Calasanti's Gendered View of Care Work," *Journal of Applied Gerontology,* Vol. 35, No. 7, July 2016, pp. 759–787.

Hooker, Stephanie A., Megan E. Grigsby, Barbara Riegel, and David B. Bekelman, "The Impact of Relationship Quality on Health-Related Outcomes in Heart Failure Patients and Informal Family Caregivers: An Integrative Review," *Journal of Cardiovascular Nursing*, Vol. 30, No. 4, Supp. 1, 2015, pp. S52–S63.

Horner-Johnson, W., K. Dobbertin, S. Kulkarni-Rajasekhara, E. Beilstein-Wedel, and E. M. Andresen, "Food Insecurity, Hunger, and Obesity Among Informal Caregivers," *Preventing Chronic Disease*, Vol. 12, October 8, 2015, p. E170.

Houlihan, N. G., "Keep Caregivers Safe: Reduce Secondary Exposure to Chemotherapy," *Oncology Nursing Forum*, Vol. 42, No. 6, November 2015, p. 695.

Huff, N. G., N. Nadig, D. W. Ford, and C. E. Cox, "Therapeutic Alliance Between the Caregivers of Critical Illness Survivors and Intensive Care Unit Clinicians," *Annals of the American Thoracic Society*, Vol. 12, No. 11, November 2015, pp. 1646–1653.

Hunt, Gail Gibson, and Susan C. Reinhard, "The Impact of America's Changing Family upon Federal and State Family Caregiving Policy," *Generations*, Vol. 39, No. 4, Winter 2015/2016, pp. 73–79.

Iris, Madelyn, Rebecca L. H. Berman, and Sarah Stein, "Developing a Faith-Based Caregiver Support Partnership," *Journal of Gerontological Social Work*, Vol. 57, No. 6–7, October 3, 2014, pp. 728–749.

Jones, Jacqueline, Carolyn T. Nowels, Rebecca Sudore, Sangeeta Ahluwalia, and David B. Bekelman, "The Future as a Series of Transitions: Qualitative Study of Heart Failure Patients and Their Informal Caregivers," *Journal of General Internal Medicine*, Vol. 30, No. 2, 2015, pp. 176–182.

Kally, Zina, Debra L. Cherry, Susan Howland, and Monica Villarruel, "Asian Pacific Islander Dementia Care Network: A Model of Care for Underserved Communities," *Journal of Gerontological Social Work*, Vol. 57, No. 6–7, 2014, pp. 710–727.

Kally, Zina, Sarah D. Cote, Jorge Gonzalez, Monica Villarruel, Debra L. Cherry, Susan Howland, Melinda Higgins, Lora Connolly, and Kenneth Hepburn, "The Savvy Caregiver Program: Impact of an Evidence-Based Intervention on the Well-Being of Ethnically Diverse Caregivers," *Journal of Gerontological Social Work*, Vol. 57, No. 6–7, 2014, pp. 681–693.

Kang, SunWoo, and Nadine F. Marks, "Marital Strain Exacerbates Health Risks of Filial Caregiving: Evidence from the 2005 National Survey of Midlife in the United States," *Journal of Family Issues*, Vol. 37, No. 18, 2016.

Kelley, Patricia Watts, Deborah J. Kenny, Deborah R. Gordon, and Patricia Benner, "The Evolution of Case Management for Service Members Injured in Iraq and Afghanistan," *Qualitative Health Research*, Vol. 25, No. 3, 2015, pp. 426–439.

Kershaw, T., K. R. Ellis, H. Yoon, A. Schafenacker, M. Katapodi, and L. Northouse, "The Interdependence of Advanced Cancer Patients' and Their Family Caregivers' Mental Health, Physical Health, and Self-Efficacy over Time," *Annals of Behavioral Medicine*, Vol. 49, No. 6, December 2015, pp. 901–911.

Kesselheim, Aaron S., Sarah McGraw, Lauren Thompson, Kelly O'Keefe, and Joshua J. Gagne, "Development and Use of New Therapeutics for Rare Diseases: Views from Patients, Caregivers, and Advocates," *The Patient: Patient-Centered Outcomes Research*, Vol. 8, No. 1, 2015, pp. 75–84.

Khodyakov, D., L. Mikesell, R. Schraiber, M. Booth, and E. Bromley, "On Using Ethical Principles of Community-Engaged Research in Translational Science," *Translational Research*, Vol. 171, 2016, pp. 52–62.

Kirk, Raymond S., and J. Kagan, *A Research Agenda for Respite Care: Deliberations of an Expert Panel of Researchers, Advocates and Funders*, Washington, D.C.: ARCH National Respite Network and Resource Center, 2015. As of January 10, 2017:
https://archrespite.org/images/docs/2015_Reports/ARCH_Respite_Research_Report_web.pdf

Kirkpatrick, J. N., K. Kellom, S. C. Hull, R. Henderson, J. Singh, L. A. Coyle, M. Mountis, E. D. Shore, R. Petrucci, P. F. Cronholm, and F. K. Barg, "Caregivers and Left Ventricular Assist Devices as a Destination, Not a Journey," *Journal of Cardiac Failure*, Vol. 21, No. 10, October 2015, pp. 806–815.

Kitko, Lisa A., *The Work of Spousal Caregiving in Heart Failure*, dissertation, State College, Pa.: Penn State University, 2014.

Knowlton, Amy R., Mary M. Mitchell, Allysha C. Robinson, Trang Q. Nguyen, Sarina Isenberg, and Julie Denison, "Informal HIV Caregiver Proxy Reports of Care Recipients' Treatment Adherence: Relationship Factors Associated with Concordance with Recipients' Viral Suppression," *AIDS and Behavior*, Vol. 19, No. 11, November 2015, pp. 2123–2129.

Koenig, H. G., B. Nelson, S. F. Shaw, S. Saxena, and H. J. Cohen, "Religious Involvement and Telomere Length in Women Family Caregivers," *Journal of Nervous and Mental Disease*, Vol. 204, No. 1, January 2016, pp. 36–42.

Krieger, Janice L., Angela L. Palmer-Wackerly, Jessica L. Krok-Schoen, Phokeng M. Dailey, Julianne C. Wojno, Nancy Schoenberg, Electra D. Paskett, and Mark Dignan, "Caregiver Perceptions of Their Influence on Cancer Treatment Decision Making: Intersections of Language, Identity, and Illness," *Journal of Language and Social Psychology*, Vol. 34, No. 6, December 2015, pp. 640–656.

Kusmaul, Nancy, and Deborah P. Waldrop, "Certified Nursing Assistants as Frontline Caregivers in Nursing Homes: Does Trauma Influence Caregiving Abilities?" *Traumatology*, Vol. 21, No. 3, 2015, pp. 251–258.

Lee, Eun-Jeong, Samantha DeDios, Camille Simonette, and Gloria K. Lee, "Family Adaptation Model for Spousal Caregivers of People with Multiple Sclerosis: Testing the Stress-Processing Theory," *Journal of Vocational Rehabilitation*, Vol. 39, No. 2, 2013, pp. 91–100.

Leggett, Amanda N., Yin Liu, Laura Cousino Klein, and Steven H. Zarit, "Sleep Duration and the Cortisol Awakening Response in Dementia Caregivers Utilizing Adult Day Services," *Health Psychology*, Vol. 35, No. 5, 2016, pp. 465–473.

Li, Andrew, Jonathan A. Shaffer, and Jessica Bagger, "The Psychological Well-Being of Disability Caregivers: Examining the Roles of Family Strain, Family-to-Work Conflict, and Perceived Supervisor Support," *Journal of Occupational Health Psychology*, Vol. 20, No. 1, 2015, pp. 40–49.

Limardi, S., A. Stievano, G. Rocco, E. Vellone, and R. Alvaro, "Caregiver Resilience in Palliative Care: A Research Protocol," *Journal of Advanced Nursing*, Vol. 72, No. 2, February 2016, pp. 421–433.

Limiñana-Gras, Rosa M., Lucía Colodro-Conde, Isabel Cuéllar-Flores, and Pilar M. Sánchez-López, "Clinical Efficacy of Psychoeducational Interventions with Family Caregivers," *Educational Gerontology*, Vol. 42, No. 1, 2016, pp. 37–48.

Lindauer, Allison, Theresa A. Harvath, Patricia H. Berry, and Peggy Wros, "The Meanings African American Caregivers Ascribe to Dementia-Related Changes: The Paradox of Hanging on to Loss," *Gerontologist*, Vol. 56, No. 4, August 2016, p. 733.

Link, Greg, "The Administration for Community Living: Programs and Initiatives Providing Family Caregiver Support," *Generations*, Vol. 39, No. 4, Winter 2015/2016, pp. 57–63.

Liu, Yin, Kyungmin Kim, David M. Almeida, and Steven H. Zarit, "Daily Fluctuation in Negative Affect for Family Caregivers of Individuals with Dementia," *Health Psychology,* Vol. 34, No. 7, 2015, pp. 729–740.

Louis, D. Burgio, E. Gaugler Joseph, and M. Hilgeman Michelle, eds., *The Spectrum of Family Caregiving for Adults and Elders with Chronic Illness,* New York: Oxford University Press, 2016.

Lundebjerg, Nancy E., and Amy M. York, "Supporting Family Caregivers Through Professional Practice: Perspectives from the Eldercare Workforce Alliance," *Generations,* Vol. 39, No. 4, Winter 2015/2016, pp. 21–27.

MacKenzie, Meredith A., Harleah G. Buck, Salimah H. Meghani, and Barbara Riegel, "Unique Correlates of Heart Failure and Cancer Caregiver Satisfaction with Hospice Care," *Journal of Pain and Symptom Management,* Vol. 51, No. 1, 2016, pp. 71–78.

MacKenzie, M. A., S. H. Meghani, H. G. Buck, and B. Riegel, "Does Diagnosis Make a Difference? Comparing Hospice Care Satisfaction in Matched Cohorts of Heart Failure and Cancer Caregivers," *Journal of Palliative Medicine,* Vol. 18, No. 12, December 2015, pp. 1008–1014.

Male, D. A., K. D. Fergus, and J. E. Stephen, "The Continuous Confrontation of Caregiving as Described in Real-Time Online Group Chat," *Journal of Palliative Care,* Vol. 31, No. 1, 2015, pp. 36–43.

Mansfield, Alyssa J., Kim M. Schaper, Alana M. Yanagida, and Craig S. Rosen, "One Day at a Time: The Experiences of Partners of Veterans with Posttraumatic Stress Disorder," *Professional Psychology: Research and Practice,* Vol. 45, No. 6, 2014, pp. 488–495. As of March 3, 2017: http://www.ptsd.va.gov/professional/articles/article-pdf/id43320.pdf

Matthews, J. T., J. H. Lingler, G. B. Campbell, A. E. Hunsaker, L. Hu, B. R. Pires, M. Hebert, and R. Schulz, "Usability of a Wearable Camera System for Dementia Family Caregivers," *Journal of Healthcare Engineering,* Vol. 6, No. 2, 2015, pp. 213–238.

McCrae, Christina S., Joseph M. Dzierzewski, Joseph R. H. McNamara, Karlyn E. Vatthauer, Alicia J. Roth, and Meredeth A. Rowe, "Changes in Sleep Predict Changes in Affect in Older Caregivers of Individuals with Alzheimer's Dementia: A Multilevel Model Approach," *Journals of Gerontology Series B: Psychological Sciences & Social Sciences,* Vol. 71, No. 3, 2016, pp. 458–462.

McCurry, S. M., Y. Song, and J. L. Martin, "Sleep in Caregivers: What We Know and What We Need to Learn," *Current Opinion in Psychiatry,* Vol. 28, No. 6, November 2015, pp. 497–503.

McIntyre, Alice, *Participatory Action Research,* Thousand Oaks, Calif.: Sage Publications, 2007.

McMillan, S. C., C. Rodriguez, H. L. Wang, and A. Elliott, "Issues Faced by Family Caregivers of Hospice Patients with Head and Neck Cancers," *ORL Head and Neck Nursing,* Vol. 33, No. 2, Spring 2015, pp. 8, 10–13.

Mendez-Luck, Carolyn A., Steven R. Applewhite, Vicente E. Lara, and Noriko Toyokawa, "The Concept of Familism in the Lived Experiences of Mexican-Origin Caregivers," *Journal of Marriage and Family,* Vol. 78, No. 3, June 2016, pp. 813–829.

Menne, Heather L., David M. Bass, Justin D. Johnson, Branka Primetica, Keith R. Kearney, Salli Bollin, Marcus J. Molea, and Linda Teri, "Statewide Implementation of 'Reducing Disability in Alzheimer's Disease': Impact on Family Caregiver Outcomes," *Journal of Gerontological Social Work,* Vol. 57, No. 6–7, 2014, pp. 626–639.

Mikesell, Lisa, "The Use of Directives to Repair Embodied (Mis)Understandings in Interactions with Individuals Diagnosed with Frontotemporal Dementia," *Research on Language and Social Interaction,* Vol. 49, No. 3, July/September 2016, pp. 201–219.

Millenaar, Joany K., Marjolein E. de Vugt, Christian Bakker, Deliane van Vliet, Yolande A. L. Pijnenburg, Raymond T. C. M. Koopmans, and Frans R. J. Verhey, "The Impact of Young Onset Dementia on Informal Caregivers Compared with Late Onset Dementia: Results from the NeedYD Study," *The American Journal of Geriatric Psychiatry,* Vol. 24, No. 6, 2016, pp. 467–474.

Miller, Edward Alan, Robert A. Rosenheck, and Lon S. Schneider, "Caregiver Burden, Health Utilities, and Institutional Service Use in Alzheimer's Disease," *International Journal of Geriatric Psychiatry,* Vol. 27, No. 4, 2012, pp. 382–393.

Mitchell, M. M., A. C. Robinson, T. Q. Nguyen, and A. R. Knowlton, "Informal Caregiver Characteristics Associated with Viral Load Suppression Among Current or Former Injection Drug Users Living with HIV/AIDS," *AIDS and Behavior,* Vol. 19, No. 11, November 2015, pp. 2117–2122.

Miyawaki, Christina E., "Sociodemographic Characteristics and Health Status of Asian, Hispanic, and Non-Hispanic White Family Caregivers of Older Adults Across Generations," *Journal of Ethnic & Cultural Diversity in Social Work,* Vol. 24, No. 4, 2015, pp. 257–279.

Monin, Joan K., Richard Schulz, and Brooke C. Feeney, "Compassionate Love in Individuals with Alzheimer's Disease and Their Spousal Caregivers: Associations with Caregivers' Psychological Health," *Gerontologist,* Vol. 55, No. 6, December 2015, pp. 981–989.

Moon, Heehyul, Aloen L. Townsend, Peggye Dilworth-Anderson, and Carol J. Whitlatch, "Predictors of Discrepancy Between Care Recipients with Mild-to-Moderate Dementia and Their Caregivers on Perceptions of the Care Recipients' Quality of Life," *American Journal of Alzheimer's Disease and Other Dementias,* Vol. 31, No. 6, 2016, pp. 508–515.

Morris, Z. S., S. Wooding, and J. Grant, "The Answer Is 17 Years, What Is the Question: Understanding Time Lags in Translational Research," *Journal of the Royal Society of Medicine,* Vol. 104, No. 12, 2011, pp. 510–520.

Morrison, Karen, Laraine Winter, and Laura N. Gitlin, "Recruiting Community-Based Dementia Patients and Caregivers in a Nonpharmacologic Randomized Trial: What Works and How Much Does It Cost?" *Journal of Applied Gerontology,* Vol. 35, No. 7, July 2016, pp. 788–800.

Nasrallah, H. A., P. D. Harvey, D. Casey, C. T. Csoboth, J. I. Hudson, L. Julian, E. Lentz, K. H. Nuechterlein, D. O. Perkins, N. Kotowsky, T. G. Skale, L. R. Snowden, R. Tandon, C. Tek, D. Velligan, S. Vinogradov, and C. O'Gorman, "The Management of Schizophrenia in Clinical Practice (MOSAIC) Registry: A Focus on Patients, Caregivers, Illness Severity, Functional Status, Disease Burden and Healthcare Utilization," *Schizophrenia Research,* Vol. 166, No. 1–3, August 2015, pp. 69–79.

National Academies of Sciences, Engineering, and Medicine, *Families Caring for an Aging America,* Washington, D.C.: National Academies Press, 2016. As of January 10, 2017: http://www.nationalacademies.org/hmd/Reports/2016/families-caring-for-an-aging-america.aspx

Nichols, Linda O., Jennifer Martindale-Adams, Robert M. D. Burns, Jeffrey M. A. Zuber, and Marshall J. Graney, "REACH VA: Moving from Translation to System Implementation," *Gerontologist,* Vol. 56, No. 1, February 2016, pp. 135–144.

Oh, Y. S., "Predictors of Self and Surrogate Online Health Information Seeking in Family Caregivers to Cancer Survivors," *Social Work in Health Care,* Vol. 54, No. 10, 2015, pp. 939–953.

Pagan-Ortiz, Marta E., Dharma E. Cortes, Noelle Rudloff, Patricia Weitzman, and Sue Levkoff, "Use of an Online Community to Provide Support to Caregivers of People with Dementia," *Journal of Gerontological Social Work,* Vol. 57, No. 6–7, 2014, pp. 694–709.

Paone, Deborah, "Using RE-AIM to Evaluate Implementation of an Evidence-Based Program: A Case Example from Minnesota," *Journal of Gerontological Social Work,* Vol. 57, No. 6–7, 2014, pp. 602–625.

Park, J. R., R. Bagatell, W. B. London, J. M. Maris, S. L. Cohn, K. K. Mattay, M. Hogarty, and COG Neuroblastoma Committee, "Children's Oncology Group's 2013 Blueprint for Research: Neuroblastoma," *Pediatric Blood Cancer,* Vol. 60, No. 6, 2013, pp. 985–993.

Patel, Bina R., "Caregivers of Veterans with 'Invisible' Injuries: What We Know and Implications for Social Work Practice," *Social Work,* Vol. 60, No. 1, January 2015, pp. 9–17.

Peng, Hsi-Ling, Rebecca A. Lorenz, and Yu-Ping Chang, "Sleep Quality in Family Caregivers of Individuals with Dementia: A Concept Analysis," *Clinical Nursing Research,* Vol. 25, No. 4, 2016, pp. 448–464.

Penwell-Waines, Lauren, Marie-Christine Rutter Goodworth, Rhonda S. Casillas, Rebecca Rahn, and Lara Stepleman, "Perceptions of Caregiver Distress, Health Behaviors, and Provider Health-Promoting Communication and Their Relationship to Stress Management in MS Caregivers," *Health Communication,* Vol. 31, No. 4, 2016, pp. 478–484.

Petty, M., "Supporting Caregivers in Caring: Empowered to Disempowered and Back Again," *Creative Nursing,* Vol. 21, No. 2, 2015, pp. 69–74.

Phillips, S. S., D. M. Ragas, N. Hajjar, L. S. Tom, X. Dong, and M. A. Simon, "Leveraging the Experiences of Informal Caregivers to Create Future Healthcare Workforce Options," *Journal of the American Geriatrics Society,* Vol. 64, No. 1, January 2016, pp. 174–180.

Piamjariyakul, U., M. Werkowitch, J. Wick, C. Russell, J. L. Vacek, and C. E. Smith, "Caregiver Coaching Program Effect: Reducing Heart Failure Patient Rehospitalizations and Improving Caregiver Outcomes Among African Americans," *Heart Lung,* Vol. 44, No. 6, November–December 2015, pp. 466–473.

Piette, John D., Dana Striplin, Nicolle Marinec, Jenny Chen, and James E. Aikens, "A Randomized Trial of Mobile Health Support for Heart Failure Patients and Their Informal Caregivers: Impacts on Caregiver-Reported Outcomes," *Medical Care,* Vol. 53, No. 8, 2015, pp. 692–699.

Piette, J. D., D. Striplin, N. Marinec, J. Chen, R. B. Trivedi, D. C. Aron, L. Fisher, and J. E. Aikens, "A Mobile Health Intervention Supporting Heart Failure Patients and Their Informal Caregivers: A Randomized Comparative Effectiveness Trial," *Journal of Medical Internet Research,* Vol. 17, No. 6, June 10, 2015, p. e142.

Pinciotti, Caitlin M., David M. Bass, Catherine A. McCarthy, Katherine S. Judge, Nancy L. Wilson, Robert O. Morgan, Andrea Lynn Snow, and Mark E. Kunik, "Negative Consequences of Family Caregiving for Veterans with PTSD and Dementia," *Journal of Nervous and Mental Disease,* 2016, pp. 106–111.

Pressler, Susan J., Irmina Gradus-Pizlo, Suzanne D. Chubinski, George Smith, Susanne Wheeler, Rebecca Sloan, and Miyeon Jung, "Family Caregivers of Patients with Heart Failure: A Longitudinal Study," *Journal of Cardiovascular Nursing,* Vol. 28, No. 5, 2013, pp. 417–428.

Ramchand, Rajeev, Nicole K. Eberhart, Christopher Guo, Eric R. Pederson, Terrance Dean Savitsky, Terri Tanielian, and Phoenix Voorhies, *Developing a Research Strategy for Suicide Prevention in the Department of Defense: Status of Current Research, Prioritizing Areas of Need, and Recommendations for Moving Forward,* Santa Monica, Calif.: RAND Corporation, RR-559-OSD, 2014. As of March 3, 2017:
http://www.rand.org/pubs/research_reports/RR559.html

Ramchand, Rajeev, Terri Tanielian, Michael P. Fisher, Christine Anne Vaughan, Thomas E. Trail, Caroline Batka, Phoenix Voorhies, Michael Robbins, Eric Robinson, and Bonnie Ghosh-Dastidar, *Hidden Heroes: America's Military Caregivers,* Santa Monica, Calif.: RAND Corporation, RR-499-TEDF, 2014. As of March 3, 2017:
http://www.rand.org/pubs/research_reports/RR499.html

Reczek, Corinne, and Debra Umberson, "Greedy Spouse, Needy Parent: The Marital Dynamics of Gay, Lesbian, and Heterosexual Intergenerational Caregivers," *Journal of Marriage and Family,* Vol. 78, No. 4, August 2016, pp. 957–974.

Rini, C., D. Emmerling, J. Austin, L. M. Wu, H. Valdimarsdottir, W. H. Redd, R. Woodruff, and R. Warbet, "The Effectiveness of Caregiver Social Support Is Associated with Cancer Survivors' Memories of Stem Cell Transplantation: A Linguistic Analysis of Survivor Narratives," *Palliative and Supportive Care,* Vol. 13, No. 6, December 2015, pp. 1735–1744.

Roddy, Sarah, Juliana Onwumere, and Elizabeth Kuipers, "A Pilot Investigation of a Brief, Needs-Led Caregiver Focused Intervention in Psychosis," *Journal of Family Therapy,* Vol. 37, No. 4, November 2015, pp. 529–545.

Romero, M. M., L. S. Flood, N. K. Gasiewicz, R. Rovin, and S. Conklin, "Validation of the National Institutes of Health Patient-Reported Outcomes Measurement Information System Survey as a Quality-of-Life Instrument for Patients with Malignant Brain Tumors and Their Caregivers," *Nursing Clinics of North America,* Vol. 50, No. 4, December 2015, pp. 679–690.

Romero, Melissa M., Carol H. Ott, and Sheryl T. Kelber, "Predictors of Grief in Bereaved Family Caregivers of Persons with Alzheimer's Disease: A Prospective Study," *Death Studies,* Vol. 38, No. 6, 2014, pp. 395–403.

Roth, D. L., P. Dilworth-Anderson, J. Huang, A. L. Gross, and L. N. Gitlin, "Positive Aspects of Family Caregiving for Dementia: Differential Item Functioning by Race," *Journals of Gerontology Series B: Psychological Sciences and Social Sciences,* Vol. 70, No. 6, November 2015, pp. 813–819.

Salgado-García, Francisco I., Jeffrey K. Zuber, Marshall J. Graney, Linda O. Nichols, Jennifer L. Martindale-Adams, and Frank Andrasik, "Smoking and Smoking Increase in Caregivers of Alzheimer's Patients," *Gerontologist,* Vol. 55, No. 5, 2015, pp. 780–792.

Sallim, A. B., A. A. Sayampanathan, A. Cuttilan, and R. Chun-Man Ho, "Prevalence of Mental Health Disorders Among Caregivers of Patients with Alzheimer Disease," *Journal of the American Medical Directors Association,* Vol. 16, No. 12, December 2015, pp. 1034–1041.

Samia, L. W., A. M. Aboueissa, J. Halloran, and K. Hepburn, "The Maine Savvy Caregiver Project: Translating an Evidence-Based Dementia Family Caregiver Program Within the RE-AIM Framework," *Journal of Gerontological Social Work*, Vol. 57, No. 6–7, 2014, pp. 640–661.

Samson, Zoe Blake, Monica Parker, Clinton Dye, and Kenneth Hepburn, "Experiences and Learning Needs of African American Family Dementia Caregivers," *American Journal of Alzheimer's Disease and Other Dementias,* Vol. 31, No. 6, 2016, pp. 492–501.

Sano, Mary, Karen Dahlman, Margaret Sewell, and Carolyn W. Zhu, "The Economics of Caring for Individuals with Alzheimer's Disease," in Steven H. Zarit and Ronda C. Talley, eds., *Caregiving for Alzheimer's Disease and Related Disorders: Research, Practice, Policy*, New York: Springer Science + Business Media, 2013, pp. 71–90.

Sav, A., S. S. McMillan, F. Kelly, M. A. King, J. A. Whitty, E. Kendall, and A. J. Wheeler, "The Ideal Healthcare: Priorities of People with Chronic Conditions and Their Carers," *BMC Health Services Research,* Vol. 15, December 14, 2015, p. 551.

Schwartz, Jack, and Leslie B. Fried, "Legal Issues for Caregivers of Individuals with Alzheimer's Disease," in Steven H. Zarit and Ronda C. Talley, eds., *Caregiving for Alzheimer's Disease and Related Disorders: Research, Practice, Policy*, New York: Springer Science + Business Media, 2013, pp. 165–179.

Schwartz, Jennifer, Matthew A. Allison, Sonia Ancoli-Israel, Melbourne F. Hovell, Ruth E. Patterson, Loki Natarajan, Simon J. Marshall, and Igor Grant, "Sleep, Type 2 Diabetes, Dyslipidemia, and Hypertension in Elderly Alzheimer's Caregivers," *Archives of Gerontology and Geriatrics,* Vol. 57, No. 1, 2013, pp. 70–77.

Shaffer, K. M., Y. Kim, M. M. Llabre, and C. S. Carver, "Dyadic Associations Between Cancer-Related Stress and Fruit and Vegetable Consumption Among Colorectal Cancer Patients and Their Family Caregivers," *Journal of Behavioral Medicine,* Vol. 39, No. 1, February 2016, pp. 75–84.

Sherman, M. D., D. A. Perlick, and K. Straits-Troster, "Adapting the Multifamily Group Model for Treating Veterans with Posttraumatic Stress Disorder," *Psychological Services,* Vol. 9, No. 4, November 2012, pp. 349–360.

Smart, C. M., and J. T. Giacino, "Exploring Caregivers' Knowledge of and Receptivity Toward Novel Diagnostic Tests and Treatments for Persons with Post-Traumatic Disorders of Consciousness," *NeuroRehabilitation,* Vol. 37, No. 1, 2015, pp. 117–130.

Smith-Johnson, B., B. L. Davis, D. Burns, A. J. Montgomery, and Z. T. McGee, "African American Wives and Perceived Stressful Experiences: Providing Care for Stroke Survivor Spouses," *ABNF Journal,* Vol. 26, No. 2, Spring 2015, pp. 39–42.

Smith-Osborne, Alexa, and Brandi Felderhoff, "Veterans' Informal Caregivers in the 'Sandwich Generation': A Systematic Review Toward a Resilience Model," *Journal of Gerontological Social Work,* Vol. 57, No. 6–7, 2014, pp. 556–584.

Stevens, Alan B., and Jennifer L. Thorud, "The Symbiosis of Population Health and Family Caregiving Drives Effective Programs that Support Patients and Families," *Generations,* Vol. 39, No. 4, Winter 2015/2016, pp. 34–38.

Stevens, L. F., T. C. Pickett, K. P. Wilder Schaaf, B. C. Taylor, A. Gravely, C. H. Van Houtven, G. Friedemann-Sanchez, and J. M. Griffin, "The Relationship Between Training and Mental Health Among Caregivers of Individuals with Polytrauma," *Behavioural Neurology,* Vol. 2015, Article ID 185941, 2015, pp. 1–13.

Sumner, L. A., D. K. Wellisch, Y. Kim, and R. L. Spillers, "Psychosocial Characteristics of Adult Daughters of Breast Cancer Patients: Comparison of Clinic and Community Caregivers Samples," *Journal of Psychosocial Oncology,* Vol. 33, No. 5, 2015, pp. 561–575.

Sun, V., M. Grant, M. Koczywas, B. Freeman, F. Zachariah, R. Fujinami, C. Del Ferraro, G. Uman, and B. Ferrell, "Effectiveness of an Interdisciplinary Palliative Care Intervention for Family Caregivers in Lung Cancer," *Cancer,* Vol. 121, No. 20, October 15, 2015, pp. 3737–3745.

Sun, Virginia, Jae Y. Kim, Dan J. Raz, Walter Chang, Loretta Erhunmwunsee, Carolina Uranga, Anne Marie Ireland, Karen Reckamp, Brian Tiep, Jennifer Hayter, Michael Lew, Betty Ferrell, and Ruth McCorkle, "Preparing Cancer Patients and Family Caregivers for Lung Surgery: Development of a Multimedia Self-Management Intervention," *Journal of Cancer Education,* 2016, pp. 1–7.

Supiano, K. P., T. C. Andersen, and L. B. Haynes, "Sudden-on-Chronic Death and Complicated Grief in Bereaved Dementia Caregivers: Two Case Studies of Complicated Grief Group Therapy," *Journal of Social Work in End-of-Life and Palliative Care,* Vol. 11, No. 3–4, 2015, pp. 267–282.

Tang, F., H. Jang, J. Lingler, L. K. Tamres, and J. A. Erlen, "Stressors and Caregivers' Depression: Multiple Mediators of Self-Efficacy, Social Support, and Problem-Solving Skill," *Social Work in Health Care,* Vol. 54, No. 7, 2015, pp. 651–668.

Tarter, Robin, George Demiris, Kenneth Pike, Karla Washington, and Debra Parker Oliver, "Pain in Hospice Patients with Dementia: The Informal Caregiver Experience," *American Journal of Alzheimer's Disease and Other Dementias,* Vol. 31, No. 6, 2016, pp. 524–529.

Taylor, B. J., L. A. Irish, L. M. Martire, G. J. Siegle, R. T. Krafty, R. Schulz, and M. H. Hall, "Avoidant Coping and Poor Sleep Efficiency in Dementia Caregivers," *Psychosomatic Medicine,* Vol. 77, No. 9, November–December 2015, pp. 1050–1057.

Thomason, M., M. Toman, and M. Potter, "Giving a Voice to Patients and Caregivers," *North Carolina Medical Journal,* Vol. 76, No. 3, July–August 2015, pp. 165–167.

Tieu, L., U. Sarkar, D. Schillinger, J. D. Ralston, N. Ratanawongsa, R. Pasick, and C. R. Lyles, "Barriers and Facilitators to Online Portal Use Among Patients and Caregivers in a Safety Net Health Care System: A Qualitative Study," *Journal of Medical Internet Research,* Vol. 17, No. 12, December 3, 2015, p. e275.

Toohey, M. J., A. Muralidharan, D. Medoff, A. Lucksted, and L. Dixon, "Caregiver Positive and Negative Appraisals: Effects of the National Alliance on Mental Illness Family-to-Family Intervention," *Journal of Nervous and Mental Disease,* Vol. 204, No. 2, February 2016, pp. 156–159.

Trevino, K. M., P. K. Maciejewski, A. S. Epstein, and H. G. Prigerson, "The Lasting Impact of the Therapeutic Alliance: Patient-Oncologist Alliance as a Predictor of Caregiver Bereavement Adjustment," *Cancer,* Vol. 121, No. 19, October 1, 2015, pp. 3534–3542.

Uphold, Constance R., Meggan Jordan, and Magaly Freytes, "Family Caregivers of Veterans: A Critical Review of the Empirical Literature and Recommendations for Future Research," in Patricia Watts Kelley, ed., *Annual Review of Nursing Research,* Vol. 32: *2014: Innovations of Care,* New York: Springer Publishing Co., 2014, pp. 155–202.

Van den Hooff, Susanne, and Anne Goossensen, "Conflicting Conceptions of Autonomy: Experiences of Family Carers with Involuntary Admissions of their Relatives," *Ethics and Social Welfare,* Vol. 9, No. 1, 2015, pp. 64–81.

Van Houtven, Courtney Harold, Joshua M. Thorpe, Deborah Chestnutt, Margory Molloy, John C. Boling, and Linda Lindsey Davis, "Do Nurse-Led Skill Training Interventions Affect Informal Caregivers' Out-of-Pocket Expenditures?" *Gerontologist,* Vol. 53, No. 1, 2013, pp. 60–70.

Votruba, Kristen L., Carol Persad, and Bruno Giordani, "Patient Mood and Instrumental Activities of Daily Living in Alzheimer Disease: Relationship Between Patient and Caregiver Reports," *Journal of Geriatric Psychiatry and Neurology,* Vol. 28, No. 3, 2015, pp. 203–209.

Walker, E. A., Y. Cao, P. A. Edles, J. Acuna, C. Sligh-Conway, and J. S. Krause, "Racial-Ethnic Variations in Paid and Unpaid Caregiving: Findings Among Persons with Traumatic Spinal Cord Injury," *Disability and Health Journal,* Vol. 8, No. 4, October 2015, pp. 527–534.

Washington, K. T., K. C. Pike, G. Demiris, D. Parker Oliver, D. L. Albright, and A. M. Lewis, "Gender Differences in Caregiving at End of Life: Implications for Hospice Teams," *Journal of Palliative Medicine,* Vol. 18, No. 12, December 2015, pp. 1048–1053.

Wiseman, J. T., S. Fernandes-Taylor, M. L. Barnes, A. Tomsejova, R. S. Saunders, and K. C. Kent, "Conceptualizing Smartphone Use in Outpatient Wound Assessment: Patients' and Caregivers' Willingness to Use Technology," *Journal of Surgical Research,* Vol. 198, No. 1, September 2015, pp. 245–251.

Wolff, J. L., J. D. Darer, and K. L. Larsen, "Family Caregivers and Consumer Health Information Technology," *Journal of General Internal Medicine,* Vol. 31, No. 1, January 2016, pp. 117–121.

Wolff, J. L., B. C. Spillman, V. A. Freedman, and J. D. Kasper, "A National Profile of Family and Unpaid Caregivers Who Assist Older Adults with Health Care Activities," *JAMA Internal Medicine,* Vol. 176, No. 3, March 2016, pp. 372–379.

Wood, Andrew W., Jessica Gonzalez, and Sejal M. Barden, "Mindful Caring: Using Mindfulness-Based Cognitive Therapy with Caregivers of Cancer Survivors," *Journal of Psychosocial Oncology,* Vol. 33, No. 1, 2015, pp. 66–84.

Woolmore-Goodwin, S., M. Kloseck, A. Zecevic, J. Fogarty, and I. Gutmanis, "Caring for a Person with Amnestic Mild Cognitive Impairment," *American Journal of Alzheimer's Disease and Other Dementias,* Vol. 31, No. 2, March 2016, pp. 124–131.

Yeh, Pi-Ming, and Margaret Bull, "Use of the Resiliency Model of Family Stress, Adjustment and Adaptation in the Analysis of Family Caregiver Reaction Among Families of Older People with Congestive Heart Failure," *International Journal of Older People Nursing,* Vol. 7, No. 2, 2012, pp. 117–126.

Zernial, Carol, "The Caregiver Teleconnection," *Generations,* Vol. 39, No. 4, Winter 2015/2016, pp. 69–72.